Brain Structure & Aging

Papers by
E. A. Wright, Jean M. Spink, Warren Andrew et al.

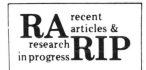

IN COOPERATION WITH THE
SMITHSONIAN SCIENCE INFORMATION EXCHANGE

Summaries of current research projects are included in the final section of this volume. Previously unpublished, these summaries were obtained from a search conducted by the Smithsonian Science Information Exchange, a national collection of information on ongoing and recently terminated research.

MSS Information Corporation
655 Madison Avenue, New York, N.Y. 10021

Library of Congress Cataloging in Publication Data
Main entry under title:

Brain structure and aging.

   1. Brain--Aging--Addresses, essays, lectures.
2. Presenile dementia--Addresses, essays, lectures.
3. Cerebrovascular diseases--Addresses, essays,
lectures. I. Wright, Eric Arthur. [DNLM: 1. Aging
--Collected works. 2. Central nervous system--
Anatomy and histology--Collected works. 3. Neuro-
chemistry--In old age--Collected works. WL300 B815
1973]
RC451.4.A5B7   618.9'76'8   73-16493
ISBN 0-8422-7175-9

TABLE OF CONTENTS

CREDITS AND ACKNOWLEDGEMENTS

Andrew, Warren, "Amitotic Division in Senile Tissues as a Probable Means of Self-Preservation of Cells," *Journal of Gerontology*, 1955, 10:1-12.

Andrew, W., "The Reality of Age Differences in Nervous Tissue," *Journal of Gerontology*, 1959, 14:259-267.

Bignami, A.; Elisabeth Beck; and H.B. Parry, "Neurosecretion-like Material in the Hindbrain of Ageing Sheep and Sheep Affected with Natural Scrapie," *Nature*, 1970, 225:194-196.

Bourne, Geoffrey H., "Changes in Dephosphorylating Enzymes in Young and Old Tissues of the Rat," *Gerontologia*, 1957, 1:50-58.

Brizzee, Kenneth R.; and Floyd A. Johnson, "Depth Distribution of Lipofuscin Pigment in Cerebral Cortex of Albino Rat," *Acta Neuropathology* (Berl.), 1970, 16:205-219.

Donahue, J. Kenneth; Robert S. Connor; and Harold W. Manner, "Observations on the Endothelial Nuclei of Certain Vertebrate Extremity Veins," *The Anatomical Record*, 1961, 139:421-427.

Epstein, Melvin H.; and Charles H. Barrows, Jr., "The Effects of Age on the Activity of Glutamic Acid Decarboxylase in Various Regions of the Brains of Rats," *Journal of Gerontology*, 1969, 24:136-139.

Hess, Arthur, "The Fine Structure of Young and Old Spinal Ganglia," *Anatomical Record*, 1955, 123:599-623.

Hughes, W., "Alzheimer's Disease," *Gerontologia Clinica*, 1970, 12: 129-148.

Prange, Jr., Arthur J.; Janice E. White; Morris A. Lipton; and A. Marcine Kinkead, "Influence of Age on Monoamine Oxidase and Catechol-0-Methyltransferase in Rat Tissues," *Life Sciences*, 1967, 6:581-586.

Spink, Jean M.; and E.A. Wright, "A Method of Making Total Nerve-Cell Counts in the Spinal Cord of Mice," *The Journal of Pathology and Bacteriology*, 1960, 79:412-416.

Sulkin, Norman M.; and Paka Srivanij, "The Experimental Production of Senile Pigments in the Nerve Cells of Young Rats," *Journal of Gerontology*, 1960, 15:2-9.

Terry, Robert D., "The Fine Structure of Neurofibrillary Tangles in Alzheimer's Disease," *Journal of Neuropathology and Experimental Neurology*, 1963, 22:629-642.

Terry, Robert D.; Nicholas K. Gonatas; and Martin Weiss, "Ultrastructural Studies in Alzheimer's Presenile Dementia," *American Journal of Pathology*, 1964, 44:269-297.

Velican, C., "Studies on the Age-Related Changes Occurring in Human Cerebral Arteries," *Atherosclerosis*, 1970, 11:509-529.

Weinbach, Eugene C.; and Joel Garbus, "Oxidative Phosphorylation in Mitochondria from Aged Rats," *The Journal of Biological Chemistry*, 1959, 234:412-417.

Wright, E.A.; and Jean M. Spink, "A Study of the Loss of Nerve Cells in the Central Nervous System in Relation to Age," *Gerontologia*, 1959, 3:277-287.

Wright, E.A.; and Jean M. Jacobs, "The Absence of Effect of X-rays on the Number of Large Nerve Cells in the Mouse Spinal Cord Two Years after Irradiation," *The Journal of Pathology and Bacteriology*, 1966, 91:613-615.

PREFACE

The importance of the central nervous system to processes of aging is of current interest to many researchers. At present, most of the basic questions remain unanswered about cellular functions in the aging brain. The present selection of articles represent a number of areas of ongoing research.

One of the most long standing beliefs about the brain is that a major general loss of neurons occurs during aging. Fortunately for humans, this belief may be more myth than reality. A number of careful studies of nerve cell population size have been carried out in the last decade which shows that gross loss of neurones is not, in fact, an inevitable consequence of aging. It is possible that some of the early studies of nerve cell loss in the human and rodent brain indiscriminantly included material with pathological lesions, such as stroke or other severe arterial occlusions, which would be expected to lead to irreparable loss of brain tissue. If significant nerve cell loss does occur during aging, it is undoubtedly regionally selective.

Structural changes in the nervous system do not appoar to involve any obvious changes in the distributions of nerve pathways. One of the most prominent lesions of aging is the accumulation of aging pigment also known as lipofuscins, Abnutztungs pigment, or wear and tear pigment. These intracellular materials have been observed to increase continuously throughout the life span and are a hallmark of normal aging. Thus far, no cellular dysfunction has been associated with their presence in brain, heart, or other tissues. The origin of these mysterious materials also remains obscure although origins from lysozomal particles have often been hypothesized.

At the metabolic level, the brain has been very little studied in terms of the effect of aging. Changes in lipid composition in the human brain could provide a basis for alterations in many cellular functions in the brain, e.g., synaptic transmitter metabolism. The scanty information available at present indicates the selective nature of age-related changes with respect to different brain regions as well as to individual enzyme reactions.

At an ultrastructural level, a number of studies employing electron microscopy have focused on the senile plaques and neurofibrillary tangles characteristic of Alzheimers disease. Although these cytopathologic changes may become frequent in the human brain during aging, a recent comparative survey of other mammals has revealed a virtual absence of senile plaques, corpora amylacose, and argyrophillic neurofibrillary tangles. It may become generally accepted that the accumulation of aging pigment is relatively unique among diverse cytological markers of aging in its apparently general incidence in non-dividing tissues. Herein, of course, lies the current dilemma of the experimental gerontologist: to find a model system for study which provides authentic characteristics of aging produced by the same underlying events in humans.

Nerve Cell Loss

A Study of the Loss of Nerve Cells in the Central Nervous System in Relation to Age

By E. A. WRIGHT and JEAN M. SPINK

The central nervous system neurones are of special interest in relation to ageing because of their undoubted importance in maintaining active life and because of the fact that when nerve cells are lost they are not replaced by division of the remaining cells. Although this last point is almost universally accepted there is some evidence that some types of cell at least show evidence of nuclear division[1]. Also neurones from adult animals have been seen to divide in tissue culture[2]. However, it seems safe to state that if nerve cell division does occur in the adult it is of little or no importance.

All methods so far used for counting nerve cells have proved to be difficult and tedious and this has led investigators to use small numbers of individuals or to use sampling techniques which are open to question. Ideally individuals should be taken from a uniform population, total nerve cell counts in defined anatomical areas should be made and the technique should be accurate and simple. Since few investigations have approached these ideal requirements we have critically reviewed some of the available data and attempted to devise a suitable technique.

Fig.1 represents graphically the results of a number of investigations relating numbers of central nervous system neurones to age in humans. In each case, except that of *Smith*, the highest unit count between 5 and 34 years has been taken as 100%.

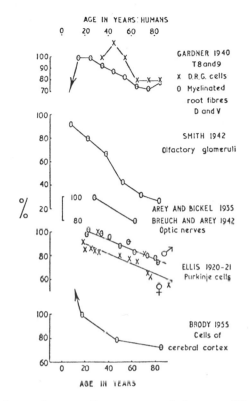

Fig. 1. Data relating total nerve cell count to age in humans. All counts have been standardized as percentages of the highest count between the ages of 15 and 34 years, except in the data of *Smith* where the counts in the newborn were taken as 100%. The arrows are directed towards the counts found at birth.

Corbin and Gardner[3] and *Gardner*[4] counted the number of myelinated fibres present in the thoracic 8th and 9th dorsal and ventral roots in over 60 cadavers. In 31 of these *Gardner* also counted the number of associated dorsal root ganglion cells. Their work is made less valuable because of the uneven distribution of subjects in the various age groups. There was one newborn infant and only 6 other individuals up to the age of 39 years. The very low counts found at birth were probably due to incomplete myelination. The uncertainty that subjects selected were from the same population having similar social and economic backgrounds also constitutes a serious criticism. An interesting finding (not shown in our figure) is that the scatter of counts between T8 and T9 is much greater in the older age groups than in the young but it is not clear on inspection

11

whether this is due to the larger numbers used in the older age groups or whether it is a true association with age. If the results can be accepted they tend to show that the greatest loss of cells occurs between the ages of 20 and 60 years, and little or no loss occurs after this.

Smith[5] cut serial sections through 205 olfactory bulbs from 121 human cadavers. He took a sample of these sections and made a numerical estimate of five degrees of integrity of each olfactory glomerulus ranging from normal to complete destruction. By adding these numerical grades he arrived at figure for each bulb. The degree of integrity was not decided upon by counting cells but by the visual impression of the degree to which the glomeruli were "motheaten". Thus the actual figures given bear a doubtful relation to numbers of nerve cells present but the general trend of the graph may have some validity. The variation between individuals increased with age, there being normal to grossly deficient individuals in every age group over 20 years of age. If the figures are accepted there appears to be a steady loss of cells throughout life.

Arey and Bickel[6] counted not less than 5% of the fibres in 6 optic nerves from individuals aged 1 to 57 years, and using the same method, *Breuch and Arey*[7] counted the fibres in 10 optic nerves from individuals with an average age of 63 years. They stated that the lower number of fibres counted in the older subjects may be a true loss with age or "may have been produced with the sample field method..." used.

Ellis[8] made estimates of the number of Purkinje cells in the cerebella of adult humans dying of various causes thought unlikely to have a direct effect on the brain cells. He attempted to estimate the number of Purkinje cells in the cerebellum by taking "equivalent unit areas" by making allowances for shrinkage and differences in size. The results show a regular fall in the number of cells per unit area with age; nearly all the female counts being lower than the male counts.

Brody[9] counted cells in the cerebral cortex of human brains. In sections of standard thickness, he also measured the depth of the cerebral cortex. Figures are given for 11 different parts of the cortex from only 4 individuals, although he reports examining 20 brains. The mean number of cells per unit area and unit volume of cortex can be computed from this data, and approximately similar results are obtained. These results are of uncertain value owing to the small number of individuals used, but if they do reflect the trend of numbers of neurones with age, they show that the loss of cells is more rapid in the early period of adult life. There are approximately twice as many cells per unit area and volume in the 2-month-old infant than in the adult; this can be accounted for in large measure by the difference in size of the infant brain compared with the adult.

Although none of these investigations is devoid of criticism they all tend to show a similar picture of nerve cell loss with age in the various parts of the central nervous system examined, and furthermore that the rate of loss is steady throughout adult life or possibly even more rapid in the earlier years. Another feature is the greater scatter of results in the older age groups. Both of these trends could be interpreted as indicating that the loss of cells was due to repeated injuries that were more frequent in the young.

When some of the data on nerve cell counts in animals is examined (fig. 2) the evidence of loss with age is less satisfactory.

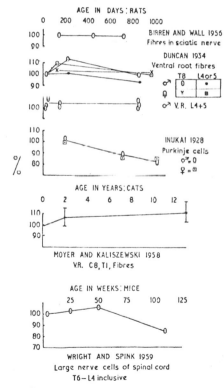

Fig. 2. Data relating total nerve counts to age in animals. In each case the counts from the youngest age group examined has been taken as 100%.

Duncan[10] counted the fibres in the ventral roots of the 8th thoracic and the 4th and 5th lumbar region in rats of various ages. The oldest animals between the ages of 850 days and 980 days do not show any appreciable loss compared with the youngest animals. *Birren and Wall*[11], counting fibres in the sciatic nerve also found no loss but their animals were only 725 days old. *Moyer and Kaliszewski*[12] examining the ventral roots of the 8th cervical and 1st thoracic segments of cats found a slight but not significant increase in the number of fibres in very old cats. The mean age of their old cats was 13 years and their oldest cat was 18 years.

Inukai[1] examined the cerebella of 6 rats; 2 young, 2 middle aged and 2 old. Their body weights were widely different. He cut serial sections of each of these cerebella and counted all the Purkinje cells in every third section. The total counts for the young, middle aged and old male rats were 547, 565 and 508×10^3 respectively and for females in the same order total counts were 425, 448 and 464×10^3. From these results it can be seen that there is no obvious relation between numbers of cells and age. Only when the figures were adjusted for surface area was a consistent and smooth loss of cells with age observed. The surface area of the "line of Purkinje cells" depended on the following factors: (a) the number of sections and the constancy of their thickness at 15μ (b) measurement of the width of the cerebellum in the fresh state after removal from the cranium and (c) measurement of the inner cortical boundary on which the Purkinje cells are situated (with a map measurer when the section is projected onto a screen). The weight of the cerebella was not recorded. The shrinkage factor calculated from (a) and (b) varied from 11.4 to 18.8%. The interpretation of these results is extremely difficult, for owing to the number and nature of the correction factors and the small number of animals used there is no certainty that the results are not due to chance. However, if one standardizes the total count to nerve cells per unit body weight or cube of the width of the cerebellum there are fewer cells in the old animals than in the young. It is clear that this type of work will have to be extended and confirmed before it can be unreservedly accepted.

Using a simple smear technique, we have counted the total number of large nerve cells in the lower spinal cord of mice of various ages.

Materials and Method

The animals were all of the BALB/C strain derived from one pair of animals which had been allowed to breed at random for 1 year before the start of the experiment. The animals remained healthy under the constant conditions of the animal house, and no epidemics occurred.

The mice in the oldest age group had received a subcutaneous injection of 0.2 ml of minced isologous embryo during the first week of life. This did not appear to have any deleterious effect on the recipients. In one of the animals used there were a few minute granules of necrotic tissue at the injection site.

The technique[13] involved the removal of the spinal column from a freshly killed mouse. The column was cut across at the intervertebral junctions, and from each of the segments thus obtained, a piece of cord was pushed out and weighed on a torsion balance. A smear of the portion of cord was made by placing it between two large coverslips which were gently pressed together and then slipped apart. The smears, after fixation in *Schaudinn*'s Fluid were transferred to alcohol, stained with haematoxylin and eosin, dehydrated, cleared and mounted. This was repeated for each segment of cord from the sixth thoracic to the fourth lumbar vertebra.

All the large nerve cells of anterior horn cell type were counted in each coverslip and the two added together to give the total number of cells in the segment of cord. Using a magnification of X 100, successive transverse sweeps of the coverslip were made from end to end. Checks on the accuracy of the counting were made by counting the same slides at different times; replicate counts were also made by a different observer. Only very occasionally was there difficulty in distinguishing the large nerve cells from other types of cell, and very few cells appeared to be distorted by this "squash" technique.

Results

Table I gives the total number of large nerve cells in the spinal cord opposite the sixth thoracic to the fourth lumbar vertebral bodies

Table I

Total Large Nerve Cell Counts in the Spinal Cord and Cord Weights (mg) in Brackets of Individual Mice of Various Ages

Age in weeks	6	25	50	110
♂	6752 (35.9)	6178 (45.4)	7197 (56.5)	5981 (65.8)
	5857 (32.0)	6097 (52.8)	7342 (62.8)	5246 (73.3)
	6130 (34.0)	5647 (50.8)	6557 (59.5)	
	6373	7745 (49.9)		
		6391 (47.1)		
Mean	6278 (34.0)	6412 (49.2)	7032 (59.7)	5614 (69.6)
♀	6428 (40.5)	6634 (52.7)	6571 (62.7)	4864 (68.5)
	5780 (37.7)	5688 (50.6)	5505 (58.6)	4225 (62.6)
	6029 (41.0)	6480 (53.9)	6117 (56.9)	5589 (66.9)
				4943 (66.0)
Mean	6079 (39.7)	6267 (52.4)	6064 (59.4)	4905 (66.0)

in the 27 mice examined. Table II shows the body weights of these mice. Figs. 3 and 4 show the number of large nerve cells, grouped into sections of three segments, at the various ages. Males and females are plotted separately so as to avoid undue influence of the

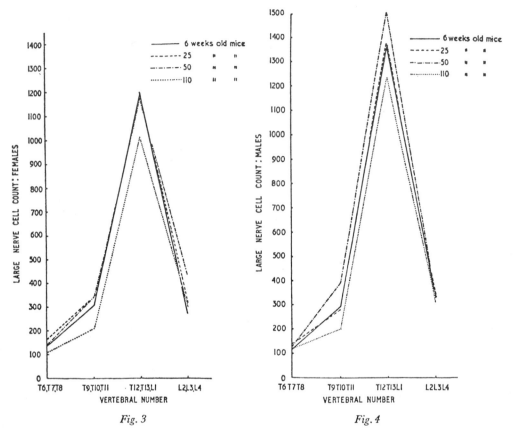

Fig. 3   Fig. 4

Figs. 3 and 4. Total large nerve cell counts in the spinal cord of BALB/C mice of various ages. For clarity the spinal segments were grouped in threes.

varying proportions of males and females. Fig. 5 shows the mean counts per mg of cord weight at each level of the cord and for each age group. In fig. 6 the mean large nerve cell counts are plotted taking the six week old animals as 100%. As there appeared to be consistently more cells in the males than in the females all the figures were calculated by taking the male and female counts separately at six weeks as 100%. The means of these percentages and the standard errors of their means could then be calculated so that com-

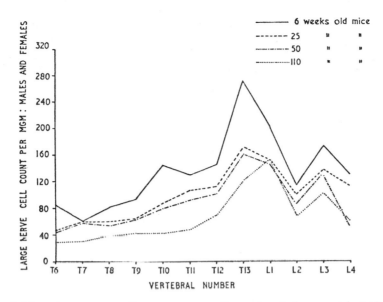

Fig. 5. Mean large nerve cell counts per mg for each spinal segment in BALB/C mice of various ages.

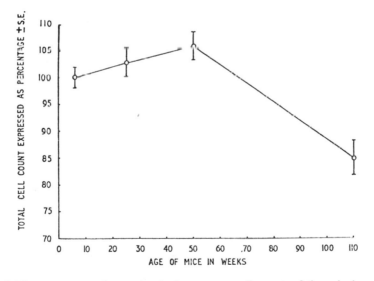

Fig. 6. The percentage changes in the large nerve cell counts of the spinal cord of BALB/C mice with age.

pensation could be made for the difference between the sexes and the numbers of each sex used.

Table II

Body Weights of Individual Mice Corresponding to Table I

Age in weeks	6	25	50	110
	12.9	20.9	28.9	25.6
♂	12.7	25.9	31.0	26.2
	12.2	24.7	28.5	
	13.6	19.7		
		20.6		
Mean	12.9	22.2	29.5	25.9
	16.3	25.3	22.6	24.9
	14.3	21.0	25.4	24.3
♀	17.2	25.4	24.8	23.0
				20.5
Mean	15.9	23.9	24.3	23.4

Discussion

Our results consistently show a smaller total number of large nerve cells in the lower spinal cord of mice in the oldest age group examined. There is probably no difference between the counts in the 6, 25 and 50-week-old even though the weights of the cord and the mouse vary by a factor of approximately two.

The population from which the mice were drawn was homogeneous as far as could be seen although the advent of some undetected environmental change or subtle genetic variation cannot be entirely excluded. The oldest mice had received an injection of minced isologous embryo a few days after birth and were therefore in this respect, different from the other groups. As a consequence of the injection they were also examined once every two to three months but this examination amounted to little more than the usual procedure of removing the mice from their cages during cleaning. If these procedures could account for the loss of nerve cells this would in itself be of considerable interest.

We believe that the technique described allows total nerve cell counts to be made accurately and simply.

Considering all the evidence from human and animal investigations it seems very likely that nerve cells are lost in the central nervous system with advancing age. The reason for this loss is not clear. The evidence shows it to vary according to the individual, the species and the type of cell under consideration: there appears to be no general law relating age with loss of cells. However, none of the work done so far on this problem, including our own, has been entirely satisfactory. Larger groups of animals from more uniform populations and more cell types need to be examined before any clear cut answers can be found. A method such as ours or that described by *Nurnberger and Gordon*[14], may overcome some of the inherent difficulties of counting nerve cells, and lead to the emergence of a more coherent picture of the relation between nerve cell death and age.

References

1. *Inukai, T.:* On the loss of Purkinje cells, with advancing age, from the cerebellar cortex of the albino rat. J. comp. Neurol. *45:* 1–31 (1928).
2. *Geiger, R. S.: In vitro* studies on the growth properties of brain cortex cells of adult individuals; in: Progress in Neurobiology II. Ultrastructure and cellular chemistry of neural tissue, pp. 83–99. Ed. *Heinrich Waelsh* (Cassell, New York 1957).
3. *Corbin, K. B.* and *Gardner, E.:* Decrease in number of myelinated fibers in human spinal roots with age. Anat. Rec. *69:* 63–71 (1937).
4. *Gardner, E.:* Decrease in human neurones with age. Anat. Rec. *77:* 529–536 (1940).
5. *Smith, C. G.:* Age incidence of olfactory nerves in man. J. comp. Neurol. *77:* 589–596 (1942).
6. *Arey, L. B.* and *Bickel, W. H.:* The number of nerve fibers in the human optic nerve. Anat. Rec. *61:* Suppl. (1935).
7. *Breuch, S. R.* and *Arey, L. B.:* The number of myelinated and unmyelinated fibers in the optic nerve of vertebrates. J. comp. Neurol. *77:* 631–665 (1942).
8. *Ellis, R. S.:* Norms for some structural changes in the human cerebellum from birth to old age. J. comp. Neurol. *32:* 1–33 (1920–21).
9. *Brody, H.:* Organization of the cerebral cortex. III. A study of ageing in the human cerebral cortex. J. comp. Neurol. *102:* 511–556 (1955).
10. *Duncan, D.:* The incidence of secondary (Wallerian) degeneration in normal mammals compared to that in certain experimental and diseased conditions. J. comp. Neurol. *51:* 197–228 (1930).
11. *Birren, J. E.* and *Wall, P. D.:* Age changes in conduction velocity, refractory period, number of fibers, connective tissue space and blood vessels in the sciatic nerve of rats. J. comp. Neurol. *104:* 1–16 (1956).
12. *Moyer, E. K.* and *Kaliszewski, B. F.:* The number of nerve fibers in motor spinal nerve roots of young, mature and aged cats. Anat. Rec. *131:* 681–700 (1958).
13. *Spink, J. M.* and *Wright, E. A.:* To be published (1959).
14. *Nurnberger, J. I.* and *Gordon, M. W.:* The cell density of neural tissues; direct counting method and possible applications as a biologic referent; in: Progress in Neurobiology II. Ultrastructure and cellular chemistry of neural tissue, pp. 100–138. Ed. *Heinrich Waelsh* (Cassell, New York 1957).

THE ABSENCE OF EFFECT OF X-RAYS ON THE NUMBER OF LARGE NERVE CELLS IN THE MOUSE SPINAL CORD TWO YEARS AFTER IRRADIATION

E. A. WRIGHT AND JEAN M. JACOBS*

THE number of neurones in the central nervous system of mammals reaches a maximum shortly after birth: in old age there is a decline in numbers (Wright and Spink, 1959). It has often been suggested that radiation advances the changes of senescence. The survival time of mice that have received a whole-body dose of 500 r. X-rays is decreased (Lindop and Rotblat, 1961); and although single doses of below 1500 r. X-rays to the central nervous system do not accelerate death, a greater loss of neurones than that normally found in later life might be expected if radiation is indeed hastening the processes of senescence.

We have therefore compared counts of large nerve cells in the spinal cord of unirradiated 2-yr-old mice with those of others of the same age that had received nearly 500 rads X-rays to the whole body when they were one month old.

MATERIALS AND METHODS

Animals. Male mice of the SAS/4 strain were exposed to 454 rads 15MeV X-rays, at a dose rate of 500 rads per minute, at the age of 30 days. For details of irradiation and survival curves of these mice see Lindop and Rotblat. Six irradiated and six sham-irradiated mice were killed at the age of 104 wk for examination of the nervous system.

Nerve cell counting. The preparation of the tissue and the staining and counting of the large nerve cells in the spinal cords of the mice have been described in detail (Spink and Wright, 1960). Essentially the procedure was to remove the spinal column from the animal and slice it across with a sharp razor blade through each intervertebral junction from T6 to L4. The cord was then pushed out, weighed rapidly and squashed between two large coverslips which were immediately fixed and stained. These two coverslips held all the cells in that segment of cord and every large nerve cell contained therein was counted.

---

* Formerly Jean M. Spink.

TABLE

TABLE

Body weight, total number of nerve cells in cord and cord weight in individual normal and irradiated mice

	Irradiated mice			Control mice		
	Body weight (g.)	Total nerve cell count in cord	Cord weight (mg.)	Body weight (g.)	Total nerve cell count in cord	Cord weight (mg.)
	35·5	7351	72·2	38·9	6647	79·6
	25·0	5939	66·0	32·6	6160	68·2
	35·1	6853	74·6	30·4	7067	76·8
	33·8	6077	70·0	31·8	7092	70·7
	32·8	6621	69·6	30·5	6282	74·5
	29·4	7012	78·0	34·1	7144	66·9
Mean . .	31·9	6642	71·7	33·1	6732	72·8
Standard error .		224			178	

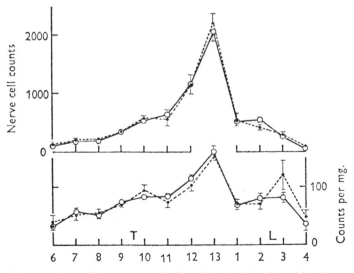

FIGURE.—Mean number of large nerve cells found in the thoracic and lumbar segments of cords of the irradiated and control mice, and nerve cell counts per mg. of cord, together with the standard errors of the means.

Control mice O———O; irradiated mice ● - - - - ●.

RESULTS

The mean numbers of large nerve cells in each segment of the cord examined in both irradiated and control animals are shown in the figure, as well as the number of large nerve cells per unit weight of cord at the various levels.

The mean total nerve count $\pm$ the standard error in the irradiated mice was 6642 ± 224 and that for the control mice 6732 ± 178 (table and figure). This result indicates that the difference is insignificant. The standard error of the difference between the two means was ± 286, thus the 95 per cent. confidence limits, taking two standard errors either side of the observed difference between means, indicate that the true count for the irradiated animals was unlikely to have been outside the limits of 9·8 per cent. below or 7·2 per cent. above the mean value observed in the control animals.

DISCUSSION

A whole-body dose of 500 r. X-rays given to mice in youth limits their lifespan (Lindop and Rotblat, 1961), but we have shown that it does not reduce the number of large nerve cells in the spinal cord. This evidence gives no support to the theory that irradiation has an ageing effect on the central nervous system. We have previously shown that there is a loss of nerve cells in the cords of old mice, thus if radiation was mimicking senescence in the central nervous system a loss of nerve cells would be expected.

Doses of radiation in the region of 2000 rads to the central nervous system cause damage that is delayed for many months (see, e.g., Russell, Wilson and Tansley, 1949), and the changes that were found could be interpreted as being due to damage to the blood vessels. With the dose of radiation given in these experiments no permanent damage to nerve cells can be demonstrated, even when the delay extends throughout almost the whole of the animals' natural lifespan.

SUMMARY

Mice were exposed to 500 rads X-rays when 30 days old. The number of large nerve cells present in the lower thoracic and lumbar cord was counted in control and irradiated mice at the age of 2 yr. No difference in cell count was found.

We are very grateful to Dr Patricia J. Lindop for her essential help in providing the irradiated and control animals and the original idea for the investigation, and we wish to thank Dr G. Rose for his advice on the statistics. This work was supported by the British Empire Cancer Fund.

REFERENCES

LINDOP, PATRICIA J., AND ROTBLAT, J.   1961.   *Proc. Roy. Soc. B*, **154**, 332.

RUSSELL, DOROTHY S., WILSON, C. W., AND TANSLEY, KATHARINE   1949.   *J. Neurol. Neurosurg. Psychiat.*, **12**, 187.

SPINK, JEAN M., AND WRIGHT, E. A.   1960.   This *Journal*, **79**, 412.

WRIGHT, E. A., AND SPINK, JEAN M.   1959.   *Gerontologia*, 3, 277.

A METHOD OF MAKING TOTAL NERVE-CELL COUNTS IN THE SPINAL CORD OF MICE

JEAN M. SPINK and E. A. WRIGHT

Although nerve cells have been observed to divide in tissue culture (Geiger, 1957) there is no evidence that cell division in the nerve cells of the central nervous system of the mammal plays any significant role once development is completed. In most mammals it appears that cell division ceases shortly after birth. As the integrity of the nerve cells is of prime importance to the well-being of the organism, and as diverse agents are known to damage and destroy these irreplaceable cells, an estimation of their numbers becomes of especial interest.

In a study of the loss of nerve cells with age (Wright and Spink, 1959) a review of some previous investigations has revealed many of the difficulties in counting neurones. The counting of nerve cells in serial sections is tedious and difficult ; counts of fibres in mixed peripheral nerves do not necessarily give the required information about the central cells ; the counting of ganglion cells in the dorsal root of the spinal cord is theoretically satisfactory but presents technical difficulties. A method recently described (Nurnberger and Gordon, 1957) involves the counting of neurone nuclei in brain tissue which has been disintegrated by shaking with glass beads. It remains to be seen whether this method will give reliable and comparable results in brains which vary widely in age and state of health.

We describe below a method of making total counts of one type of nerve cell in the spinal cord of mice.

23

Procedure

The mouse is killed with coal gas ; it is immediately pinned out and opened up from the dorsal aspect. The muscle overlying the vertebral column and ribs is dissected away, and the whole vertebral column from the base of the skull to the level of the iliac processes is removed. The ribs are cut off about 0·5 centimetres either side of the column.

The last thoracic vertebra is identified and a cut is made with a sharp scalpel above the neural spine at the intervertebral junction ; a similar cut is made at the intervertebral junction of the first lumbar vertebra. The last thoracic vertebra is then removed, the cord pushed out of the vertebral foramen with a blunt probe and weighed on a torsion balance.

The portion of the cord is placed between two coverslips ($2 \times \frac{7}{8}$ in.), which are pressed together gently but sufficiently firmly to spread the cord evenly over the coverslips, before slipping them slowly apart. The smears are fixed immediately in Schaudinn's fluid (concentrated aqueous mercuric chloride, 2 parts, alcohol, 1 part) for one hour.

In a similar manner, smears are made of each segment from the twelfth to the sixth thoracic vertebræ, and then from the first to the fourth lumbar vertebræ. Nerve fibres surrounding the cord from the third and fourth lumbar vertebræ are removed.

The smears are transferred from Schaudinn's fluid to absolute alcohol for one hour, and after treatment with iodine and sodium thiosulphate to remove mercuric chloride deposits, they are stained with Harris's hæmatoxylin for three minutes. After decolorisation in acid alcohol for a few seconds, the smears are washed in running water for at least fifteen minutes and lightly counterstained with eosin. The smears are washed, dehydrated in alcohol, cleared in xylol and mounted on slides with Canada balsam.

The coverslips may be numbered on the back with glass marking ink before making the smears, and stained back to back in groups of twelve pairs at a time.

Counting. All the large nerve cells of anterior horn cell type in each smear are counted at a $\times 100$ magnification. The field is moved over the width of the coverslip and then adjusted laterally until a fixed point noted on the extreme left of the field has been moved to the extreme edge of the right side of the field. Cells partially in the field on the left are included, those on the right excluded. A hand tally counter may be used.

The large nerve cells are easily distinguished with the slight degree of over-staining with hæmatoxylin. Only very occasionally are cells damaged in making the smears and in many cases these are still recognisable as large nerve cells.

Accuracy. To check the accuracy of the counting technique, replicate counts were made on nine pairs of smears, selected at random but including counts from various parts of the cord.

The difference between replicate counts was expressed as a percentage of the mean of the counts. The mean of the percentage difference was 4·24, and the standard deviation of this mean was 3·65. At a probability of 0·05, the fiducial limits were 4·24-8·13. This means that in 19 cases out of 20, the percentage difference would lie between 0 and 12 per cent. with a mean of 4·24.

An obvious source of error lies in the division of the cord into segments. However, from inspection of the cord weights from a typical example shown in fig. 1, it can be seen that a fairly smooth curve can be obtained.

In investigations to which this technique has been applied the total number of cells was used, and only inaccuracies at the extreme ends of the cord would then be of significance. Also, a more representative statistic of the over-all

24

technique was obtained by taking the total count. Applying the same statistical method used above to the series of counts instead of individual counts, i.e. expressing the mean difference between all the counts as a percentage of the mean of the average counts, it was found that 19 times out of 20 the percentage difference would lie between 0 and 7·68, with a mean of 3·13.

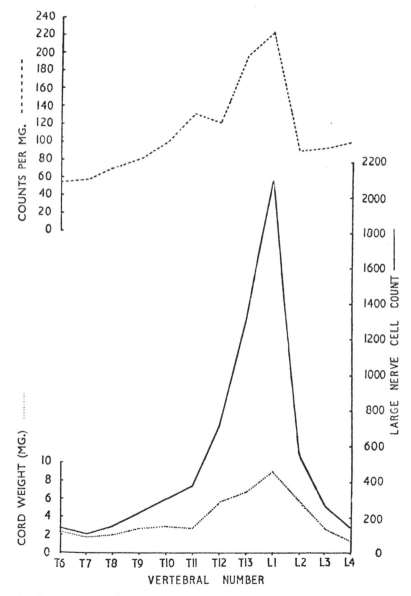

FIG. 1.—Large nerve cell counts, cord weights and counts per unit weight for each spinal segment from a young adult male BALB/C mouse.

Results

A typical example of the nerve-cell counts and weights of the spinal cord segments from a 6-month-old male BALB/C mouse is shown in fig. 1. The counts per unit weight of cord indicate a greater density as well as an absolute increase at the lumbar enlargement. The rise in counts per unit weight in the third and fourth lumbar segments is due to the fact that the ventral and dorsal roots forming the beginnings of the cauda equina were removed.

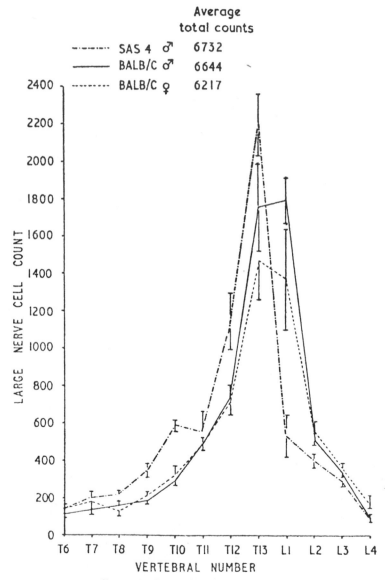

Fig. 2.—Large nerve cell counts for each spinal segment and average total counts from male SAS 4, and male and female BALB/C mice.

26

Fig. 2 shows nerve-cell counts and total counts from 6 male SAS 4, and 8 male and 6 female BALB/C mice. The difference between the two strains is small, but there is a more significant difference between the sexes. The SAS 4 strain of mice shows a slightly different distribution of cells from that of the BALB/C strain.

The nerve cells show little distortion and remain well separated from each other.

Discussion

We believe that this technique offers several advantages over other methods used to count neurones, e.g. Inukai (1928) and Smith (1942).

The selection of a fixed anatomical area avoids the necessity for making complicated calculations for variations in volume ; total cells are counted so that no statistical adjustments for sampling methods are necessary ; the preparation of smears is far less tedious and time-consuming than the production of serial sections ; fewer slides are used and cells are easier to count ; the use of a simple routine strain is an obvious advantage.

The method has been applied to a study of the loss of nerve cells in relation to age (Wright and Spink, 1959) and to an investigation into the effect of irradiation on nerve cells.

Summary

A new technique is described for making counts of large nerve cells from smears of spinal cord segments in mice. Some typical results from different strains and sexes are shown.

We are grateful to Miss M. Weinstock for her help with statistical calculations. The SAS 4 mice were kindly supplied by Dr P. J. Lindop.

NEURONE COUNTS IN MOUSE SPINAL CORD

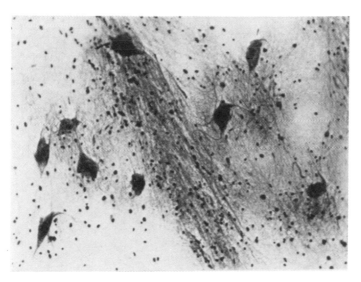

FIG. 3.—Smear with 9 large nerve cells. Hæmatoxylin and eosin. × 100.

REFERENCES

GEIGER, R. S. . . . . 1957. *In* Ultrastructure and cellular chemistry of neural tissue (Progress in Neurobiology, II), ed. by H. Waelsch, *London, Toronto, etc.*, p. 83.

INUKAI, T. . . . . 1928. *J. Comp. Neurol.*, **45**, 1.

NURNBERGER, J. I., AND GORDON, M. W. 1957. *In* Ultrastructure and cellular chemistry of neural tissue (Progress in Neurobiology, II), ed. by H. Waelsch, *London, Toronto, etc.*, p. 100.

SMITH, C. G. . . . . 1942. *J. Comp. Neurol.*, **77**, 589.

WRIGHT, E. A., AND SPINK, JEAN M. 1959. *Gerontologia*, **3**, 277.

AMITOTIC DIVISION IN SENILE TISSUES AS A PROBABLE
MEANS OF SELF-PRESERVATION OF CELLS

WARREN ANDREW, Ph.D., M.D.

IN one of our earlier investigations (1) we studied the effects of fatigue on the Purkinje cells of the cerebellum in mice of different ages. In this study we noted that the senile animals, both control and experimental, showed some Purkinje cells which were binucleate. In a later study on alterations of the Golgi apparatus with age in mice (3), binucleate Purkinje cells again were noted in all of the old animals and also a number of cells with the nucleus in the shape of a dumbbell or a horseshoe. Stages in a process of amitotic division of the nucleus were strongly indicated by these figures.

Similar phenomena were observed by Inukai (21) in the cerebellum of albino rats. In animals of 200 days some cells with elongated nuclei and 2 nucleoli were found, and in 3 senile rats of 730, 1017, and 1085 days, the presence of multiple nuclei was noted.

Whether or not the phenomena of amitotic division and binuclearity of the Purkinje cell in old age are found only in rodents has not been settled to our complete satisfaction. There are some indications that the condition is not found as a feature of senility in man (2) although occurring in certain pathologic conditions (4).

Presented at the Sixth Annual Scientific Meeting of the Gerontological Society, Inc., August 25-27, 1953, San Francisco.
This investigation has been aided by a grant from the Josiah Macy, Jr. Foundation.

In the present investigation the problem of the occurrence of amitosis in the Purkinje cells of old mice has been re-examined. In addition, observations have been made on preparations of human liver tissue.

SURVEY OF PREVIOUS STUDIES IN AMITOSIS

Mechanism of Amitosis.—According to the classical descriptions of amitosis the nucleolus generally is drawn out at an early stage and then divided into equal parts. Meanwhile the nucleus is elongating into the form of an hour-glass. The nucleus then becomes constricted and divides, generally into equal parts, each with 1 of the 2 new nucleoli. Such a process was called by Flemming (14) amitosis or direct nuclear division, in contrast to the process of mitosis or indirect nuclear division which he described in detail in 1882.

A type of amitosis which is of particular interest is described as "not rare" for many plant cells. The nucleus is divided by the formation of a very delicate fissure without a constriction of any kind and without separation of the 2 daughter nuclei. Later a diaphragm of separation between 2 halves of the nucleus is formed and only then do the 2 daughter nuclei separate. This type of division, seen many times in nature, is the type described as occurring in cells of *Spirogyra* as a result of the action of ether.

Lettré (24) discusses some of the chemical differences which probably determine the basic distinction between amitosis and mitosis. During cell division, as in the cleavage of the sea-urchin egg, the total quantity of nucleic acid is not increased, yet the thymonucleic acid (DNA), present only in small quantity at the beginning of mitosis, increases in amount at the expense of the ribonucleic acid (RNA), so that a formation of DNA from RNA apparently is occurring.

30

This fact is related to the occurrence of amitosis. The nuclear membrane of the resting or interphasic nucleus is a protein membrane upon which are heaped up the nucleic acids or nucleotides. In the separation of the chromatin the nucleic acid is removed from the nuclear membrane, causing it to lose the character of a nucleoproteid membrane and making it, as simply a protein membrane, subject to solution by the action of proteolytic ferments. This, according to Lettré, is the ordinary course of chemical events in mitotic division. If, however, the nucleic acids are not removed from the membrane, it cannot be dissolved. We then obtain the picture of amitotic division.

Occurrence of Amitosis.—Amitotic division accompanied or followed by division of the cell body is not common but yet is not extremely rare if a broad survey of the biologic field is made. Ranvier (30) in 1875 described such division in the lymphocytes of the amphibian, Axolotl, which were observed in a moist chamber. Ranvier even described the observation as simple enough for use as a class exercise. Arnold (7) confirmed his finding.

Clara (10) has described the process of amitotic division in the human liver. His specimens came from a rather heterogeneous group, with the cause of death not known in every case, so that it is difficult to draw conclusions concerning the relationship between age and the occurrence of amitosis from his material. His important conclusion from the study of livers from 20 subjects, however, is that amitosis does occur. He describes and pictures the process of division of the nucleolus in amitosis, a particular observation which seems to us to preclude any contention that he was in reality looking at figures of abnormal mitotic division. As in our own studies, he has found amitosis to be a relatively rare occurrence, but one the reality of which cannot be denied. In an 80 year old person there were 16 constricted nuclei among 5123 cells, while in a 36 year old person there were 15 constricted nuclei out of 3758 cells.

Wassermann (37) also describes amitotic division of the nuclei of liver cells. More recently Schiller (33) has described interesting observations on this phenomenon, again in human liver. He believes that such division serves as a method of freeing nuclei from the large inclusions which often appear in them since one of the daughter nuclei always will lack this "encumbrance."

Rzhevutskaia (32) described what may seem at first consideration to be a very surprising instance of amitosis. He found amitotic division in the spinal ganglion cells of puppies 5 to 7 days old giving rise not only to new nuclei but to new nerve cells. His pictures seem very convincing. The new cells are at least at first contained within the same capsule and may show perfectly parallel, flattened edges of the cell bodies.

Observations on living cells in tissue cultures have yielded some data on the occurrence of amitotic division. Holmes (20) saw amitotic division of the nuclei in ectodermal cells of the adult frog without cytoplasmic division. Kreibich (22) described amitosis of epithelial cells of the epidermis and cornea of the pig. Lewis and Webster (26), after prolonged watching, observed a single case of direct cleavage of the nucleus without division of the cytoplasm in an epithelioid giant cell. They believed, however, that amitosis is the regular manner of formation of multinucleate giant cells in cultures of lymph nodes, and found all stages of amitosis in them. In embryonic chick liver grown in vitro Lynch (27) observed direct division of the nucleus without cell division.

In general, observations of amitosis in living cells are rather rare, and Lewis and Lewis (25) reported that they had never seen amitosis in cultures of embryonic chick material. Nevertheless, they stated (p. 146): "There are so many indications of the process, however, especially in older cultures, that it is hard to believe it does not occur more frequently than the observations on living cells would indicate." Various stages of fragmentation and budding of nuclei also occur in many older cultures. Cells with such nuclei often are degenerate, as evidenced by extensive vacuolation, granular rather than flamentous mitochondria, and a reduction in the total mitochondrial content.

Cowdry (11), in a study of the mitochondria during cell division in chick embryos (fixed material) reported 907 of the cells studied as being in mitosis, 93 in apparent amitosis.

In the field of tissue culture studies, Bucher (9) described amitosis as a rare occurrence in normal cultures of fibroblasts but readily observed in cultures which were fixed 48 hours after the end of the action of colchicine upon them. In such amitoses, he said, there is no trace of formation of chromosomes, while the nuclear membrane and the nucleoli, except for division of the latter, remain absolutely intact. There is therefore no possible confusion with pseudoamitosis, a confusion against which Politzer (29) has cautioned.

In both the older and more recent literature, then, descriptions of amitotic division in a variety of cells are not lacking.

Significance of Amitosis.—It was observed by Nathansohn (28) that cells of *Spirogyra* which had undergone amitosis as a result of the action of ether were capable of ordinary mitosis when flaments were placed in water. This fact tends to discount the "sentence of death" which some cytologists have sought

33

to pronounce on all cells undergoing amitosis. Häcker (15) similarly found that the cells of embryo cephalopods which had undergone amitosis could again resume mitotic division.

Amitosis has been described as the common method of reproduction in some cells which hardly can be considered degenerate. Thus Regaud (31) has described this as the mode of division of the cells of Sertoli in the testis.

It is true, however, that amitotic division of nuclei seems to be less often concerned with multiplication of cells than with the reproduction of nuclei within an individual cell to increase the nuclear surface and thus aid in metabolic activity when "excessive" growth has occurred or when unfavorable conditions threaten the life of the cell. Dogiel (12) described it as occurring among the cells of the superficial layers in the epithelium of the urinary bladder. Such a process apparently occurs in the formation of some types of giant cells, in the follicle cells of eggs both among invertebrates and vertebrates, and in the embryo sac of phanerogamic plants. Other important instances of amitosis are in the division of nuclei in developing skeletal muscle when fibrillae are beginning to be formed and in the syncytial tissue of the placenta (18).

The amitotic process generally occurs in cells with large nuclei. Bucher (9) believes that it is caused not by the direct action of colchicine but through a modification of the internal organization of the nucleus (probably polyploidization) and that the process through the production of 2 or 3 nuclei in a cell restores the proper ratio between nuclear surface area and volume required for the metabolism of the cell.

Our citation of a number of the earlier authors does not mean that we believe that their conclusions should be accepted without considering the very real possibilities of misinterpretation. In view of more recent studies, however, including our own findings in senile tissues, we believe that these earlier descriptions should not be cursorily dismissed as obviously in error.

PRESENT STUDIES

MATERIAL AND METHODS

For the present investigation we have gone back to the study of the cerebellum of the mouse, the type of material in which our first observations on amitotic division were made. We have attempted, first, to ascertain the general picture of this process in regard to the frequency of its occurrence in animals of different ages. Second, we have attempted to study carefully the individual stages in the process to see whether it occurs in a perfectly constant manner, or if variations occur, what they may be. Third, we have given attention to the manner, if any, in which the cytoplasmic body, with its distinctive form in the Purkinje cells, may be affected by the nuclear division.

As a subsidiary to the study of the nerve cells in the senile mouse, we have initiated observations on the brains of starved animals, in which we thought that the tendency to amitosis might be increased. While this phase of the work is in an initial stage, chiefly because of the lack of more senile animals, we present some data from the study to date.

Lastly, as a cell type for comparison, we have examined the liver of a number of human subjects to see if we could confirm earlier reports of amitotic division in the hepatic cell.

The mice used in our study of the Purkinje cells comprise 12 animals of the C57 Black strain. The ages ranged from 4 to 6 weeks up to 23 to 25 months (table 1). The mice

35

Table 1. Data on the Cerebella of C57 Black Mice at Different Ages, Based on the Study of 1000 Purkinje Cells in Each Animal.

Age and Sex	Binucleate Cells	Cells with Nuclei of Altered Form	Cells with Nuclei of Normal Form but with 2 Nucleoli	Cells with Aberrant Shape of Cell Body
4-6 week Female	0	3	3	0
11-12 week Female Fed	1	5	0	0
11-12 week Female Starved	2	9	4	0
6-10 month Male	1	9	0	2
6-10 month Male	3	11	0	1
6-10 month Male	5	8	0	2
18-20 month Female	4	6	2	1
18-20 month Female	0	5	2	5
18-20 month Female	6	4	2	2
18-20 month Female	6	8	1	0
23-25 month Female Fed	20	32	0	3
23-25 month Female Starv'd	40	32	2	9

had been kept for some weeks in clean plastic cages in our own animal room after reaching us from the Jackson Memorial Laboratory. They were fed on Purina dog chow, containing all of the essential nutritional factors, and had ample supplies of water.

The ages of 4 of the mice, 2 of the 11 to 12 weeks and 2 of the 23 to 25 months, made them well-paired for an examination of the possible effect of starvation on the frequency of occurrence of the binucleate condition. Although the number of older animals was small, it was considered worth while to employ one of them in this way since our earlier work (3) already had shown that binucleate cells are increased in number in old age.

Ten of the animals, therefore, were sacrificed while in a normal, well-fed condition. Two of the animals, 1 of the 11 to 12 week ones, and 1 of the senile, 23 to 25 month ones, were starved for one week, having sufficient water but no food during this time, and then sacrificed.

The brains of all animals were divided into right and left halves. The right halves were used in making Nissl preparations, the left in special preparations such as the DaFano silver impregnation for cell form and Golgi apparatus or the Altmann's acid aniline fuchsin method for mitochondria with Regaud fixation. The present report is chiefly on the Nissl preparations. The half of the brain used for this purpose was fixed in alcohol, cleared in xylol, infiltrated and embedded in paraffin, sectioned sagittally at 4 μ, and stained with cresyl violet.

The method used in studying amitotic phenomena was to follow the border of the granular layer of the cerebellum until observation on 1000 Purkinje cells in each animal had been made.

The studies on human liver were carried out on 10 autopsy specimens from subjects with varied causes of death. The object

TABLE 2. AUTOPSY SUBJECTS USED IN A STUDY OF AMITOSIS IN THE HUMAN LIVER.

Age and Sex	Race	Cause of Death
50 year Female	Negro	Pulmonary embolism
55 year Male	Negro	Acute congestive heart failure, pulmonary tuberculosis
64 year Female	Negro	Metastatic hypernephroma of right kidney
67 year Male	White	Cerebellar herniation
70 year Female	White	Purulent bronchitis
71 year Female	White	Thrombosis, left internal capsule
72 year Female	White	Coronary thrombosis
80 year Male	Negro	Peritonitis, pulmonary infarction, pneumonia
81 year Male	Negro	Uremia, fever of central nervous etiology
96 year Male	White	Acute cardiac failure, coronary occlusion

here was not a quantitative study but an exploration of the tissue for figures of amitotic division. The subjects studied are listed in table 2.

OBSERVATIONS

Cerebellum of Mice.—A study of table 1 shows that binucleate Purkinje cells seem to be present, although in very small numbers, at a relatively early age. While none was found in the youngest mouse, the 11 to 12 week control animal showed 1 out of 1000 cells, the starved animal only 2. The 6 to 10 month animals, representing a somewhat heterogeneous group in relation to age, showed from 1 to 5 binucleate cells each.

In the 18 to 20 month old animals, the number of binucleate cells observed per thousand varied from 0 to 6. In the senile animals the normally fed mouse showed 20, the starved one 40 such cells. A Purkinje cell in the process of amitotic division is presented in figure 1.

The appearance of the binucleate cells was not the same in every instance nor in every animal. The usual arrangement, and that seen almost without exception in the binucleate cells in the senile animals, was the presence of 1 nucleus at each side of the cell body, as shown in figure 2. Another arrangement was that in which there was 1 nucleus in its normal position and another, generally smaller nucleus between it and the portion of the cell body from which the apical dendrite arises. This latter condition was true in 6 out of the 9 binucleate cells found in the 6 to 10 month animals, but seldom seen in the senile mice.

Generally a nucleolus could be found in both nuclei and very frequently a nucleolus was seen in each half of a constricted nucleus as though the division of this body were complete before the nuclear division. In some cases, however, we were unable to see any nucleolus in 1 nucleus, even in studying serial sections. Such seemed to be particularly the case with the apical nuclei of the 6 to 10 month mice which we have mentioned.

The cells with nuclei of altered form represented chiefly constricted or lobed nuclei. It was not always possible to say whether such nuclei indicate a process of amitotic division, although in many instances such a process seemed strongly indicated or practically certain (fig. 1).

It was interesting to note that constriction and lobation did not seem to be the only method by which a nucleus may form 2 daughter nuclei even within the rather

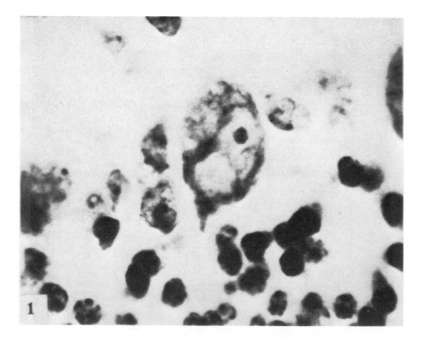

Fig. 1. Purkinje cell in the cerebellum of a 702 day old mouse. The nucleus is constricted in the process of amitotic division. Cresyl violet. X1822.

homogeneous type of the Purkinje cells. In a number of instances a delicate line of division, a split or furrow, seemed to divide the parent nucleus without its changing shape. It will be recalled from our survey of previous studies in amitosis that this type of division has been described in plant cells, and Bucher (9) has observed it in fibroblasts. We have seen it also in the salivary glands of senile rats (5, 6) and in the lesions of senile keratosis.

We were interested in the third item in table 1, namely, the number of cells with nuclei of normal form but showing 2 nucleoli, because we wished to know whether there was evidence of a prior division of the

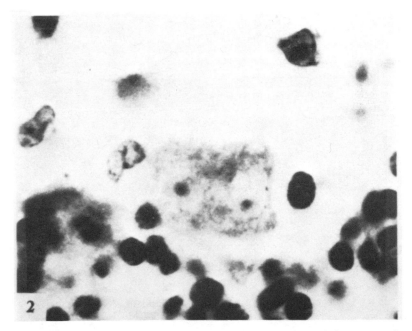

FIG. 2. Large, binucleate Purkinje cell in the cerebellum of the same animal. Each nucleus contains a prominent nucleolus. The voluminous cytoplasm is so disposed as to give a form to the cell which is very unusual for this particular cell type. Cresyl violet. X1822.

nucleolus before the nuclear form was altered. In other parts of the nervous system in rodents and some other animals, as in the spinal ganglia, the presence of 2 or more nucleoli in a nucleus is not uncommon. In the Purkinje cells, however, as our table shows, this is an unusual condition, with only 16 out of the 12,000 cells showing 2 nucleoli in the same section. There seemed to be no relation between this condition and age nor between it and the number of cells with 2 nuclei or in process of amitotic division.

The last item in table 1 is one concerning the shape of the cell body and involves the question to what extent the cytoplasm may share in the division process. A number of

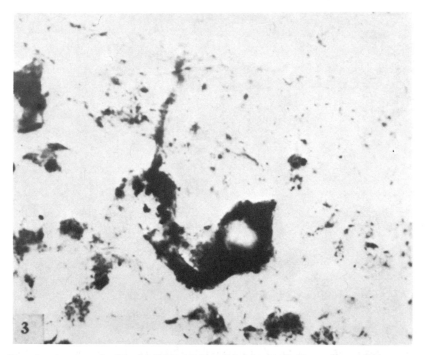

FIG. 3. Apparently "double" Purkinje cell in the cerebellum of a senile mouse which had been deprived of food for several days. The cell seems to have undergone a fission extending through its body and a short way along the axon. Da Fano silver preparation X1522.

cells with 2 nuclei were obviously of greatly increased transverse diameter (fig. 2). Some of these depart widely from the classical somewhat pear-shaped picture of the Purkinje cell. In classifying cells as having an aberrant shape of the cell body we have tried to list only those which are conspicuously aberrant, and the numbers given were not large. Some individual cases, however, were so suggestive of a tendency of the two portions of the cell to separate from each other, particularly in our senile starved animal, that we examined carefully a number of slides prepared by silver impregnation (Da Fano) which delineates the cell shape better than do the Nissl preparations. We present

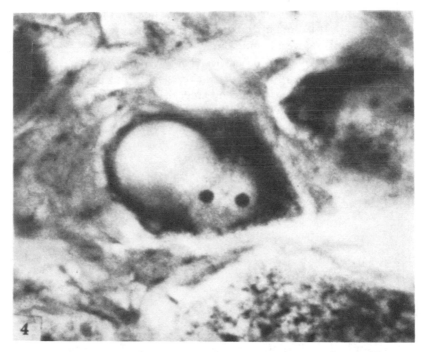

FIG. 4. Cell from a spinal ganglion of a senile dog, 12 years of age. The very large vacuole on the left represents a stage in fatty degeneration. The binucleolate condition is not uncommon in ganglion cells, but this degenerate cell seems to show a tendency to duality of the nucleus itself. Preparation courtesy of Dr. N. Sulkin. Cresyl violet. X1822.

figure 3 as an example which has been rather convincing to us of the possibility of cytoplasmic division occurring and continuing through the cell body and into the basal axon, leaving 2 "cells" attached to a common axon which is of a Y-shape. As to the functional capacity of such a morphologic arrangement, we would find it difficult to comment.

Human Liver.—The survey of liver tissue from 10 human autopsy subjects has yielded figures which we believe definitely are amitotic. These figures are not numerous and thousands of cells often must be examined to yield one. With the heterogeneous features of the subjects studied, we would not be able to relate these figures closely to the age of the individual but the fact of the real occurrence of this process we believe can hardly be doubted (figs. 5, 6, and 7). It is hoped that studies on laboratory animal material may help to relate the occurrence of amitosis in the liver in a more definite way to the aging process, as has been done for nervous and for other glandular tissues in such animals.

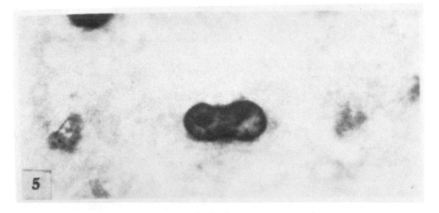

FIGS. 5-7 are from the liver of a 72 year old white woman, who died of coronary thrombosis. There was a history of diabetes mellitus in this subject.

FIG. 5. Amitotic division of a small nucleus in the liver. The 2 daughter nuclei here will be approximately equal in size and each contains a nucleolus. X1822.

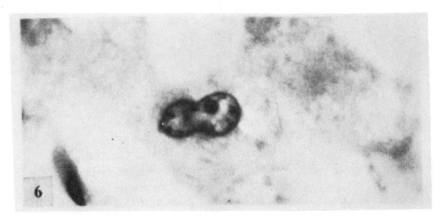

FIG. 6. Amitotic division of a small nucleus, in which the resulting nuclei apparently will be of somewhat unequal size. X1822.

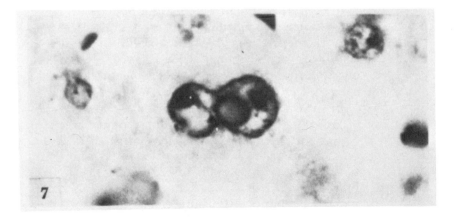

FIG. 7. Amitotic division of a large nucleus in the liver. This nucleus contains one of the inclusion bodies common in senile livers and this body occupies a portion of the constriction. X1822.

Our studies on senile tissues, including particularly gland cells (submandibular and parotid glands) and nerve cells, show that the process of amitosis occurs in such tissues, not in a large number of cells but in a consistent manner not seen in the same tissues in younger animals. The result of the amitotic division of the nucleus probably is for the most part the creation of binucleate cells which are better able to survive under the conditions prevailing in the senile tissues.

In the nervous system, a definite tendency to degeneration and death of individual cells has been shown to occur in old age.

Hodge (19) found a 25 per cent loss of Purkinje cells in a man of 92 years as contrasted with one of 47 years. Harms (17) found 16 Purkinje cells in a senile ape (*Pithecus fascicularis*) for every 41 such cells in a young ape of the same species. In an 80 year old woman this author found 5 or 6 Purkinje cells, of which only 2 were apparently functional, for every 20 in a young person.

Ellis (13) gave figures on numbers of Purkinje cells in a given area of cerebellum as follows: 823 in a man 42 years old; 591 in a man 65; 500 in a man 79; 462 in a man 94; and 445 in a man 100.

In the dog Harms (16) found 31 Purkinje cells in a 2 year old animal; 20 in a 14 year old one; and 10 in one 17 years old, in comparable areas.

In the rodents, Spiegel (34) found the loss of Purkinje cells in senile guinea-pigs to be as high as 40 per cent. The degeneration of the cells, according to him, takes place in serial fashion, involving as many as 20 to 25 cells in a row on a given section. Inukai (21) found the number of Purkinje cells in the rat at over 1000 days to be 79.6 per cent of that at 200 days and in the male, 81.6 per cent. Our own findings on the cerebellum of the

46

mouse show a comparable degree of loss of cells in this species in senility.

Truex (35) has shown that fatty degeneration of individual cells in sensory ganglia in man is responsible for the loss of many neurons after middle age. Truex and Zwemer (36) studied this process in the Gasserian ganglion and in spinal ganglia in old cats and rats and found it to be widespread in this animal material also.

Studies on parts of the nervous system other than the cerebellum and sensory ganglia show evidence of cell loss both by counts on cells (Brody on the cerebral cortex, 8) and by degenerative changes seen in them (Kuntz, on the autonomic ganglia, 23). An illustration of a binucleolate spinal ganglion cell with fatty degeneration from a senile dog is presented in figure 4.

It therefore seems clear that in the nervous system of the senile animal or man we are dealing with a population of cells which shows a rather high mortality and in which probably many or all of the cells are having to combat unfavorable conditions of existence. Under such conditions the process of amitotic division may be a not unimportant one in preserving cells which otherwise would be totally lost to the organism.

The question as to whether amitotic division ever results in the formation of new cells in senile tissues is difficult to answer. In the nervous system, where such a happening might seem least likely to occur because of the highly differentiated nature of the cells, we find some definite changes in form of the cell body in cases where 2 nuclei have been formed by amitosis and in rare instances (fig. 3) the cytoplasm seems to share in the division.

It is hoped that further studies using the silver methods for delineation of cell form may add to our knowledge of the potentialities of amitotic division.

47

SUMMARY

Observations on the tissues of senile animals give evidence of an occurrence of true amitotic division, particularly in the salivary glands and in portions of the nervous system.

A re-examination of the amitotic process as it occurs in the Purkinje cells has shown differences in detail as to the way in which the nucleus may divide. A participation of the cytoplasm in the division in some cases is strongly suggested by the present study.

Survey of autopsy sections of human liver yields figures of amitotic division of nuclei.

REFERENCES

1. Andrew, W.: The Effects of Fatigue Due to Muscular Exercise on the Purkinje Cells of the Mouse, with Special Reference to the Factor of Age. *Ztschr. f. Zellforsch. u. mikr. Anat., 27:* 534-554, 1938.
2. Andrew W.: The Purkinje Cell in Man from Birth to Senility. *Ztschr. f. Zellforsch. u. mikr. Anat., 28:* 292-304, 1938.
3. Andrew, W.: The Golgi Apparatus in the Nerve Cells of the Mouse from Youth to Senility. *Am. J. Anat., 64:* 351-375, 1939.
4. Andrew, W.: Origin and Significance of Binucleate Purkinje Cells in Man. *Arch. Path., 28:* 821-826, 1939.
5. Andrew, W.: Age Changes in the Salivary Glands of Wistar Institute Rats with Particular Reference to the Submandibular Glands. *J. Gerontol., 4:* 95-103, 1949.
6. Andrew, W.: Age Changes in the Parotid Glands of Wistar Institute Rats with Special Reference to the Occurrence of Oncocytes in Senility. *Am. J. Anat., 85:* 157-198, 1949.
7. Arnold, J.: Ueber Theilungsvorgänge an den Wanderzellen, ihre progressiven und regressiven Metamorphosen. *Arch. f. mikr. Anat., 30:* 205-310, 1887.
8. Brody, H.: Age Changes in the Human Cortex (Abstract). *Anat. Rec., 115:* 289, 1953.
9. Bucher, O.: Divisions Nucléaires Amitotiques dans des Cultures de Fibrocytes Après Administration de Colchicine. *Acta anat. 4:* 60-67, 1947-1948.
10. Clara, M.: Untersuchungen an der menschlichen Leber. II. Teil. Über die Kerngrössen in den

48

Leberzellen. Zugleich über Amitose und über das Wachstum der "stabilen Elemente." *Ztschr. f. mikr.-anat. Forsch., 22:* 145-219, 1930.

11. Cowdry, E. V.: The Relations of Mitochondria in Cells Multiplying by Mitotic and Amitotic Division (Abstract). *Anat. Rec., 8:* 102, 1914.

12. Dogiel, A. S.: Zur Frage über das Epithel der Harnblase. *Arch. f. mikr. Anat., 35:* 389-404, 1890.

13. Ellis, R. S.: Norms of Some Structural Changes in the Human Cerebellum from Birth to Old Age. *J. Comp. Neurol., 32:* 1-33, 1920.

14. Flemming, W.: *Zellsubstanz, Kern und Zellteilung.* F. C. W. Vogel, Leipzig, 1882.

15. Häcker, V.: Die Reifungserscheinungen. *Ergebn. Anat. u. Entwcklngsgesch., 8:* 847-922, 1898.

16. Harms, W.: Morphologische und experimentelle Untersuchungen an alternden Hunden. *Ztschr. f. Anat. u. Entwcklngsgesch., 71:* 319-382, 1924.

17. Harms, W.: Alterserscheinungen im Hirn von Affen und Menschen. *Zool. Anz. 74:* 249-256, 1927.

18. Hintzsche, E.: Beobachtungen über die Kerngrösse menschlicher Zellen. *Ztschr. f. mikr.-anat. Forsch., 39:* 45-56, 1935.

19. Hodge, C. F.: Changes in Ganglion Cells from Birth to Senile Death. Observations on Man and Honeybee. *J. Physiol., 17:* 129-134, 1894.

20. Holmes, S. J.: The Behavior of the Epidermis of Amphibians When Cultivated Outside the Body. *J. Exper. Zool.,* 281-294, 1914.

21. Inukai, Tetsuo: Loss of Purkinje Cells with Age in the Albino Rat. *J. Comp. Neurol., 45:* 1-33, 1928.

22. Kreibich, C.: Zellteilung in kultivierter Haut und Kornea. *Arch. f. Dermat. u. Syph., Orig., 120:* 925-930, 1914.

23. Kuntz, A.: Histological Variations in Autonomic Ganglia and Ganglion Cells Associated with Age and Disease. *Am. J. Path., 14:* 783-799, 1939.

24. Lettré, H.: Neuere Ergebnisse der Chemie der Kern- und Zellteilung. *Zentralbl. Gynäk, 72:* 1851-1863, 1950.

25. Lewis, W. H., and M. R. Lewis: Behavior of Cells in Tissue Cultures. In E. V. Cowdry, editor, *General Cytology, The University of Chicago Press*, Chicago, 1924.

26. Lewis, W. H., and L. T. Webster: Giant Cells in Cultures from Human Lymph Nodes. *J. Exper. Med., 33:* 349-360, 1921.

27. Lynch, R. S.: The Cultivation in Vitro of

Liver Cells from Chick Embryos. *Am. J. Anat.*, *29:* 281-312, 1921.

28. Nathansohn, A.: Physiologische Untersuchungen über amitotische Kernteilung. *Jahrb. wiss. Botan.*, *35:* 48-79, 1900.

29. Politzer, G.: Pathologie der Mitose. *Protoplasma-Monographien*, *7:* Borntrager, Berlin, 1934.

30. Ranvier, L.: *Traité Technique d'Histologie.* F. Savy, Paris, 1875.

31. Regaud, C.: Quelques Details sur la Division Amitotique des Noyaux de Sertolie chez le Rat. Sort du Nucléoli. Deux Variétés d'ámitose: Équivalence ou Nonéquivalence des Noyaux-Fils. *Verhandl. d. anat. Gesell.*, *14:* 100-124, 1900.

32. Rzhevutskaia, O. P.: (Amitotic division of nerve cell in cerebrospinal ganglia in the dog). *Doklady Akad. nauk. SSSR.*, *87:* 483-484, 1952.

33. Schiller, E.: Kerneinschlüsse und Amitose. *Ztschr. f. Zellforsch. u. mikr. Anat.*, *34:* 356-361, 1949.

34. Spiegel, A.: Über die degenerativen Veränderungen in der Kleinhirnrinde im Verlauf des Individualzyklus vom Cavia cobaya Marcgr. *Zool. Anz. 79:* 173-182, 1928.

35. Truex, R. C.: Morphological Alterations in the Gasserian Ganglion Cells and Their Association with Senescence in Man. *Am. J. Path.*, *16:* 255-268, 1940.

36. Truex, R. C., and Zwemer, R. L.: True Fatty Degeneration in Sensory Neurons of the Aged. *Arch. Neurol. & Psychiat.*, *48:* 988-995, 1942.

37. Wassermann, F.: Die Amitose, in "Wachstum und Vermehrung der lebendigen Masse," in: *Handbuch der mikroskopischen Anatomie des Menschen*, I /2, edited by W. v. Möllendorff. Julius Springer. Berlin, 549-583, 1929.

Aging Pigment

Depth Distribution of Lipofuscin Pigment in Cerebral Cortex of Albino Rat*

KENNETH R. BRIZZEE and FLOYD A. JOHNSON

Summary. The proportion of neuron somata occupied by lipofuscin pigments was determined at 20 relative depth levels throughout the depth of cerebral cortex (area 3) through the use of an integrating ocular and application of the Chalkley (1943) "hit" method.

The proportion of the neuron soma volume occupied by autofluorescent granules was calculated from the above data. The highest (peak) values were observed in lamina Vb ($23^0/_0$-aged, $13^0/_0$-middle age, and $6^0/_0$-young adult). Mean values for the entire depth of cortex increased from $3^0/_0$ in 100 day rats to $6^0/_0$ in 400 days and $13^0/_0$ at $630-700$ days. The *proportional* increase in the relative volume of cell soma occupied by lipofuscin pigment from young adulthood to old age was greatest in lamina III, followed closely by lamina II.

Ultrastructural studies of neurons in lamina V of cerebral cortical area 3 of young adult (150 day) and very aged (1200 day) albino rats revealed that electron-dense pigment bodies in neuron somata tended to increase in amount and size with increase in age of the animals. These changes were accompanied by changes in gross configurations and internal structure of the pigment bodies and a tendency to congregate in groups within the perikarya. Similar changes, although more variable, were observed in pigment accumulation within perineuronal glial cells.

Key-Words: Lipopigment, Neuronal and Glial — Ultrastructure — Fluorescence Microscopy — Ageing.

This investigation was supported by AEC contract *AT-(40-1)-3832*.

A recent investigation of the amount and distribution of lipofuscin pigment in the cerebral cortex of the albino rat (Brizzee, Cancilla, Sherwood and Timiras, 1969) revealed a marked increase, from young adulthood to old age, in the amount of pigment per neuron soma in both the superficial (lamina II) and deep region (lamina V). The proportional increase per unit cell volume was greater in the superficial than in the deeper region, although the absolute amount of pigment remained higher in the latter region. It has been suggested by some investigators that the accumulation of lipofuscin in neurons may have an appreciable physiologic effect and may even result in a loss of cells (Samorajski, Keefe and Ordy, 1964; Samorajski, Ordy and Keefe, 1965). The resolution of the question as to the possible physiologic and behavioral effects of lipofuscin accumulation in neurons of animals at any age level must depend initially upon an accurate analysis of the relative, as well as absolute, changes in pigment mass in neurons and glia in response to various environmental conditions (e.g. radiation exposure). The present report constitutes a continuation of our recent quantitative histological studies on lipofuscin pigments (Brizzee, Cancilla, Sherwood, and Timiras, 1969) and is concerned with an analysis of the absolute and proportional accumulation with age of lipofuscin at various depth levels in the rat cerebral cortex.

Materials and Methods

Three male and two female albino rats of the Sprague-Dawley strain at each of three age levels (100 days, 400 days, and 630−700 days) were fixed by perfusion with a two-stage perfusion procedure employing Elliott's "B" solution and 10% neutral formalin (Cammermeyer, 1960). Dehydration of the brain tissues was carried out through graded ethyl alcohols, and the tissues were cleared in normal butyl alcohol, embedded in Paraplast, sectioned at 6μ, and mounted unstained in a low-fluorescence mounting medium. The sections were examined with blue-light fluorescence at a wave length of about 420 mμ, the light source being a high pressure mercury vapor burner (Osram HBO-200). The light beam was filtered through a BG 38 heat absorbing filter and a BG-12 exciter filter. A UG 1 barrier filter was inserted between a Leitz phasecontrast fluorescence $90 \times$ oil immersion objective and $10 \times$ ocular on a Leitz Ortholux binocular microscope.

The proportion of the oil immersion field area occupied by autofluorescent pigment bodies was determined with the use of an integrating (measuring point) eyepiece in which a number of fine crosslines were distributed in a pattern designed to provide random sampling of the fields. Sixteen such crosslines (points) were counted at each of 20 equally spaced, successive depth levels (Fig. 1) in the submolecular cortex in cerebral cortical area 3 (Krieg, 1946) in every section. Eight such traverses from the superficial level (superficial border of lamina II) to the deep level (deep border of lamina VI) were made in each section, and counts were made in four sections in each brain. Thus, five hundred and twelve points were counted at each of the twenty cortical depth levels in each brain. "Hits" were recorded (Chalkley, 1943) wherever the fine crosslines (points) of the measuring point ocular coincided with autofluorescent bodies located in neuron somata in which a neuron nucleus or a portion of such a nucleus could be identified unequivocally. It is of importance to emphasize that the level of focus was the middle depth level, or middle focal plane of each section, and only the autofluorescent granules which were clearly in focus in that plane were counted. Following this procedure an accurate comparison of changes in relative amounts of autofluorescent pigment in neurons of young adult as compared with aged brains was obtained. No attempt was made to determine the proportion of autofluorescent bodies in neuron fragments not associated with clearly defined neuron nuclear structures, because of the possibility of including autofluorescent bodies in neuroglia in such counts.

In order to determine the proportion of the mean oil immersion field area occupied by neuron somata, similar "point" counts were carried out on sections prepared as described above but stained with the buffered thionin method at pH 4.5. "Hits" were recorded wherever the fine crosslines (points) of the measuring point ocular coincided, at the middle depth focal plane, with neuron somata in the thionin preparations.

In order to provide an accurate measurement of the 20 relative cortical depth levels, each binocular microscope was equipped with a two-dial mechanical stage (x and y axes) reading in 10 μ units. Only the dial representing the "y" axis was used for this study.

To demonstrate the ultrastructural characteristics of the pigments in young adult and very aged animals, albino rats of the Sprague-Dawley strain were sacrificed at 100, 150, 300, and over 1200 days[1] of age. The brains were fixed by perfusion with 2.5% glutaraldehyde buffered at pH 7.4 with sodium phosphate buffer (Karlsson and Schultz, 1965 and Schultz and Karlsson, 1965), postfixed in 1% osmium tetroxide, and embedded in Epon 812. Sections 1 μ thick were examined under a phasecontrast microscope to select cortical lamina V from blocks of cerebral cortical area 3 for final thin sectioning. The ultrathin sections were doublestained with magnesium uranyl acetate and lead citrate and examined with an RCA EMU 3G electron microscope.

Results

The presence of autofluorescent granules in laminae III and V of cerebral cortex in young (100 day) and aged (630—700 day) animals is illustrated in Figs. 2 and 3. In the young adults a few granules were observed in most neurons in all laminae, having essentially a random, scattered distribution in the perikaryon as illustrated for lamina III in Fig. 2 A. The marked accumulation of the pigment granules in cells of the same type in an aged animal is shown in Fig. 2 B. In Fig. 3 A the relative amount and general distribution of the pigment material in large pyramidal cell neurons of lamina V of a young adult animal is shown. In Fig. 3 B the massive accumulation of the pigment with age in a pyramidal cell neuron is illustrated. In cytoarchitectonic laminae II, IV and VI the general appearance and cellular distribution of the pigment was similar to that shown in Figs. 2 and 3. However, in neurons of

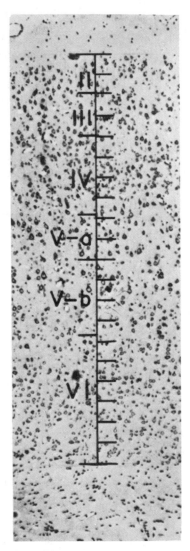

Fig. 1. Photomicrograph of transverse section of cerebral cortex in area 3 showing cytoarchitectonic laminae II through VI and corresponding 20 relative depth levels throughout depth of submolecular cortex. Thionin, 6 μ ×83

---

1 The 1200 days old animals were obtained from the laboratories of Dr. Denham Harmon, Department of Biochemistry, University of Nebraska College of Medicine.

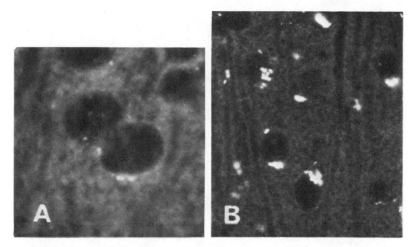

Fig.2A and B. Photomicrographs of unstained sections under blue light fluorescence illustrating autofluorescent granules in neuron somata of lamina III of cerebral cortex. A Young adult ×1684; B Aged ×1000

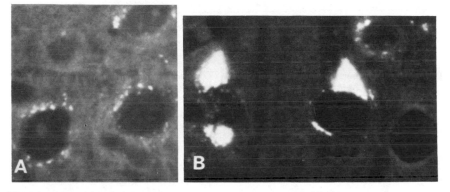

Fig.3A and B. Photomicrographs of unstained sections under blue light fluorescence illustrating autofluorescent granules in neuron somata in lamina V of cerebral cortex. A Young adult ×1500; B Aged × 1050

lamina VI in aged brains the pattern as well as amount of pigment appeared somewhat more variable than in the other laminae. In 400 day animals the pigment accumulation in various laminae varied considerably but generally appeared intermediate in amount between that observed in the young adult and aged groups.

The proportion of the cerebral cortical tissue occupied by neuron somata at the various depth levels in the three age groups is illustrated in Fig.4. While the mean values obtained for the aged group tend to be lower than the young adult group, the mean differences between groups for the 20 levels was not significant ($p > 0.05$). It was observed from the figure that the values average about

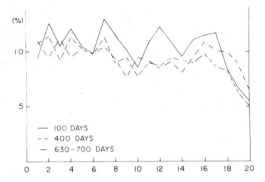

Fig.4. The mean proportion (%) of oil immersion field in submolecular cerebral cortex occupied by neuronsomata in thionin-stained sections

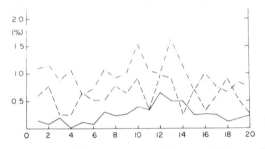

Fig.5. The mean proportion (%) of oil immersion field occupied by autofluorescent granules located in neuron somata in submolecular cerebral cortex in unstained preparations

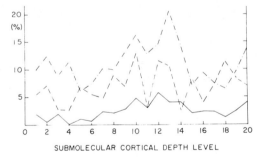

SUBMOLECULAR CORTICAL DEPTH LEVEL

Fig.6. The mean proportion (%) of neuron somata occupied by autofluorescent granules in submolecular cerebral cortex

11% in the outer half of the cortex, and decrease somewhat in the deeper half with lowest values (about 5%) observed in the deep part of the multiform layer at relative depth levels 19 and 20.

The proportion of the mean oil immersion field occupied by autofluorescent granules within the neuron somata at the 20 relative depth levels is illustrated in Fig.5. While the values are low (mainly less than 0.5% in young adults and

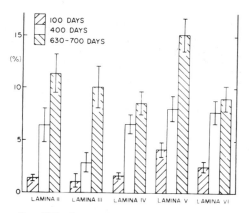

Fig. 7. The mean proportion (%) of neuron somata occupied by autofluorescent granules in individual cytoarchitectonic laminae

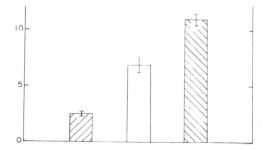

Fig. 8. The mean proportion (%) of neuron somata occupied by autofluorescent granules throughout submolecular cerebral cortex in area 3

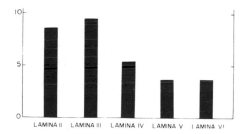

Fig. 9. The proportional increase in the amount of neuron somata occupied by autofluorescent granules in cytoarchitectonic laminae of submolecular cerebral cortex from young adulthood (100 days) to old age (630—700 days)

below 2.0% in aged) the differences between all age groups, considering the mean values for all of the 20 depth levels, were significant ($p < 0.05$). The curve for the aged group revealed a significant decline ($p < 0.05$) from the most superficial levels (1—4; external granular layer and external pyramidal layer) to slightly deeper levels (5—9; internal granular layer) and peak values at levels 10, 13, and 14 (internal pyramidal layer). This pattern was less evident in the younger

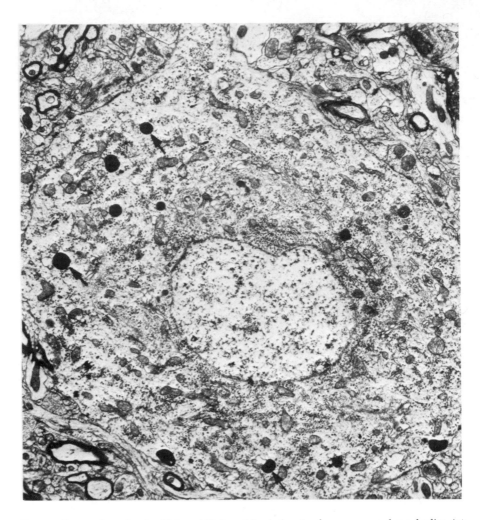

Fig. 10. Neuron from lamina V in a 150 day-old rat showing homogeneous dense bodies (at arrows) scattered at random in the perikaryon. × 6100

age groups, though peak values were found in the internal pyramidal layer in all groups.

The proportion of neuron somata occupied by lipofuscin pigment material (Fig. 6) was calculated from the data illustrated in Figs 4 and 5. The trends observed in this graph were similar to those seen in Fig. 5, but the peak areas were more definite, the highest value (23%) being observed at depth level 13 in the internal pyramidal layer (lamina V b).

The mean value for proportion of neuron somata occupied by the pigment bodies in individual subcortical cytoarchitectonic laminae (II through VI) is shown in Fig. 7. The highest values were observed in lamina V at all age levels,

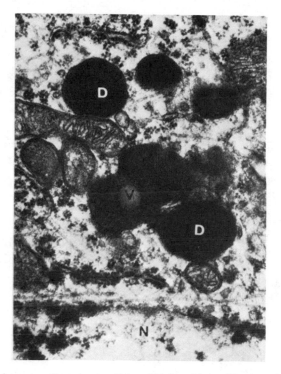

Fig. 11. Portion of a neuron from lamina V in a 100 day-old rat. The dense bodies (*D*) are of a granular homogeneous structure. A small vacuole (*V*) is present in a body near the nucleus (*N*). ×31,800

and the difference between the value in lamina V and the lamina with the next highest value (II) in aged animals was significant at the 0.01 level. The mean value for the proportion of neuron somata occupied by the pigment bodies for the entire depth of submolecular cortex at the three age levels is shown in Fig. 8. The values increased from 3% in 100 day rats to 6% in 400 day and 13% in 630—700 days. From this data it appears that the increase in amount of lipofuscin per unit volume of cerebral cortical neuron soma occurred virtually as a straight line function in the tissues studied.

Despite the higher peak values and absolute amount of lipofuscin pigment observed in the internal pyramidal lamina, the *proportional increase* in amount of neuron somata occupied by lipofuscin pigment from young adulthood to old age was significantly greater in the external granular and external pyramidal laminae than in any other cortical lamina (Fig. 9).

Electron micrographs revealed that the distribution of dense bodies within neuron somata corresponded with that of the auto-fluorescent bodies seen under blue light excitation. These dense bodies were identical to those described by Samorajski, Keefe, and Ordy, (1964); Samorajski, Ordy, and Keefe (1965); Samorajski, Ordy, and Rady-Reimer (1968), as lysosomes and lipofuscin.

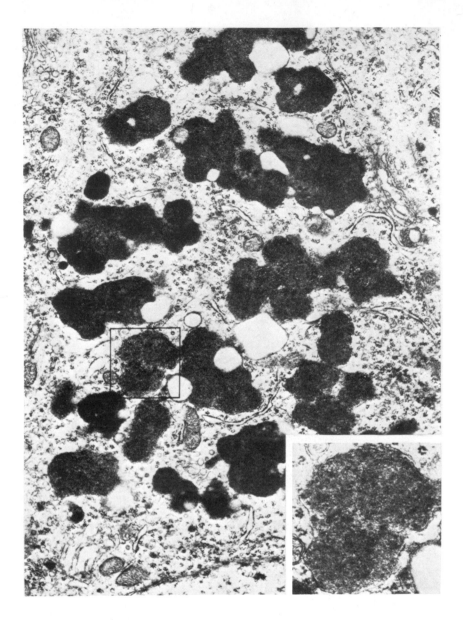

Fig. 12. Portion of a neuron from lamina V in a 1200 day-old rat. The lipofuscin pigments are clustered at one pole of the nucleus. ×14,700. Inset shows lobed structure observed in many of the pigment bodies. ×32,550

Most of the neurons examined from the adult subjects (100 and 150 days of age) showed a few dense bodies distributed randomly in the perikarya (Fig. 10). These dense bodies tended to be homogeneous, round to ovoid, and were bounded by single limiting membranes. An occasional body contained a small vacuole

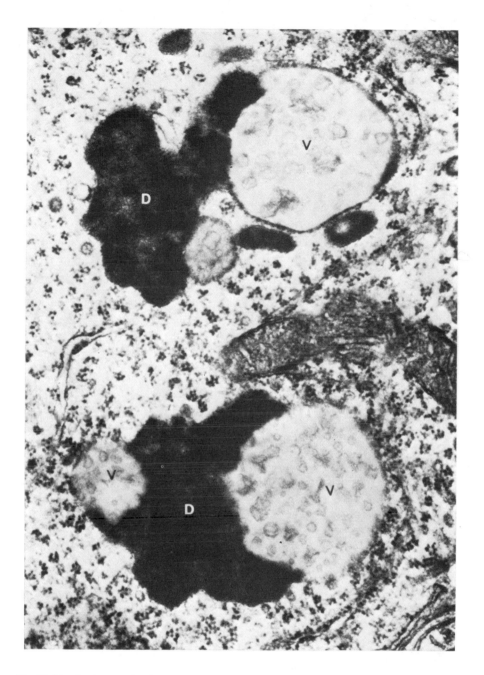

Fig. 13. Lipofuscin granules from a neuron in a 1200 day-old rat showing dense (*D*) and vacuolar (*V*) components. The vacuoles contain vesicle-like structures. ×43,000

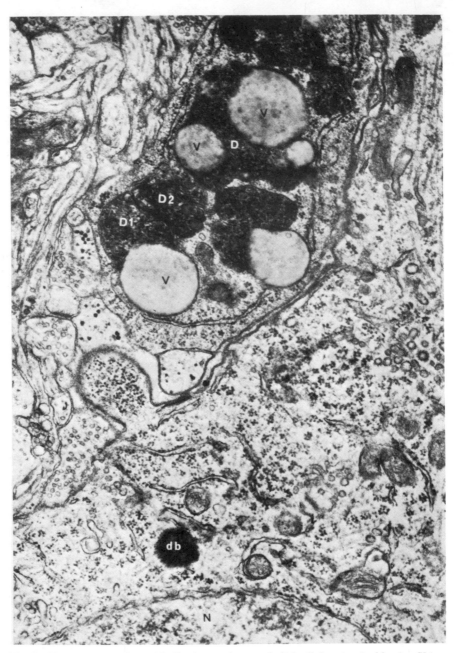

Fig. 14. Heterogeneous pigment bodies in a perineuronal glial cell from cortical lamina V in a 300 day-old rat. The bodies consist of dense (D) and vacuolar (V) components. The internal structure at D1 is mostly granular whereas the adjacent lobe (D2) contains larger rounded particles. Each lobe (D1 and D2) appears to be contained by its own limiting membrane. A dense body (db) is also present in the neuron perikaryon near the nucleus (N). ×25,300

(Fig.11). Neuron somata of the intermediate age subjects (300 days of age) showed approximately the same amount of scattered dense bodies but in addition an increased number of cells showed larger, more irregularly shaped bodies, presumed to be lipofuscin pigments, congregated in groups. These bodies were more complex and more variable in structure, having vacuolar and dense components. The dense components sometimes showed dark and light patches and lamellations.

The oldest subjects (1200 days) showed the largest amounts of pigments. In addition to a few small homogeneous dense bodies scattered randomly in the perikarya, most neurons showed clusters of large, heterogeneous lipofuscin pigments. These clusters were most often located at the base of the apical dendrites of pyramidal neurons (Fig.12) although in many neurons pigment clusters were observed at the base of axonal hillocks or elsewhere within the perikarya. The variable structure described for the intermediate aged subjects was more pronounced in the aged subjects, and many of the vacuolar components contained small vesicle-like structures (Fig.13).

Dense bodies were also observed within perineuronal glial cells. These were more varied in amount and structure than those within neurons (Fig.14). These bodies, like their neuronal counterparts, consisted of dense and vacuolar components. The vacuolar elements differed little from those observed in neuron somata, and the dense elements were similarly varied in form. However, the internal structure of the dense elements was more heterogeneous, as can be seen in Fig.14. The dense matrix of the lobe (D1) containing the large vacuole consisted mostly of coarse granules and a few larger rounded particles. The adjacent lobe (D2) consisted mostly of the larger rounded particles and a much smaller amount of the granular material. Each of the two lobes appeared to be contained by its own single limiting membrane. In some specimens, curved bands with myelin-like periodicity were observed.

Discussion

Comparing data obtained in this investigation with those seen in our previous study (Brizzee, Cancilla, Sherwood and Timiras, 1969) we noted that maximal values for proportion of neuron somata occupied by lipofuscin granules is lower (5%) in neurons of lamina V of young adults of the present group than in the corresponding group in the previous study (12%). However, maximal mean values for neurons of lamina V in aged animals in the present study (15%, Fig.7) are only slightly lower than in the previous investigation (18%), and the peak value in lamina V in the present group (23%) was a little higher than in the earlier investigation.

In both young adult (100 days) and aged (630—700 days) animals in lamina II, the proportion of neuron somata occupied by autofluorescent granules was appreciably lower in the present study (2%) and (12%) than in the earlier investigation (8%) and (18%). The *proportional* increase in the amount of pigment per unit neuron volume, however, was greater in the tissues studied in the current investigation than in the initial study, in both lamina II and lamina V. A new finding in the present study was the observation that the *proportional* increase in this parameter from young adulthood to old age was greater in lamina III than in any other cytoarchitectonic lamina.

A number of investigators including Einarson and Telford (1960a, b) and Miyagishi, Takahata and Iizuka (1967) have demonstrated that lipofuscin pigments, structurally indistinguishable from those observed in aged animals were observed in nerve cells of young animals subjected to diets deficient in vitamin E. It has also been demonstrated (Sulkin, 1959), and (Sulkin and Srivany, 1960) that lipofuscin formation is accelerated in animals subjected to chronic anoxia or acetanalid administration. Sulkin (1959) demonstrated that lipofuscin pigment could be induced in dogs of only 3 months of age and was enhanced in certain stress conditions regardless of the age of the animals. In our present study, conditions of diet and housing were standardized for animals in all age groups. Thus, although we recognize the validity of the observations of the investigators cited above, it appears that the differences in absolute amounts as well as relative concentrations and rate of accumulation of lipofuscin pigments in various strata of the cerebral cortex in our own preparations, were definitely age-related.

Ultrastructural studies of cerebral cortical lamina V corroborated the results of fluorescence microscopy with regard to the distribution and accumulation of pigments within neuron somata. The variations observed in the amounts and structure of dense bodies in neuron somata, and the even wider variations within perineuronal glial cells, indicate a need for studying the ultrastructure of dense bodies in both neuron and glia somata in all cytoarchitectonic laminae. This would broaden the basis for evaluating the relationship of lysosomes and lipofuscin pigments to cell physiology. It would also be expected to shed more light on the role of satellite cells in neuronal physiology.

Many investigators have presented evidence to implicate lysosomes in the formation of lipofuscin pigments. Samorajski, Keefe, and Ordy (1964) suggested that lipofuscin pigments are altered lysosomes. Some of the pigments in our material were clearly lobed (Fig. 12 inset) suggesting coalescense of several rounded bodies, believed to be of lysosomal origin, to form one lipofuscin pigment. This structural detail was also observed in a number of pigments in perineuronal glial cells (Fig. 14).

Our present ultrastructural study revealed that some perineuronal glial cells in subjects of all ages contained heterogeneous dense bodies presumed to be lipofuscin pigments. These were rare in the young adults (100—150 day) and more numerous in the intermediate (300 day) and aged (1200 day) specimens. However, pigment bodies were completely absent from electron micrographs of many perineuronal satellite cells, even in aged subjects. This may indicate an absence of pigments in some cells, but in others the plane of sectioning probably excluded them from the ultra-thin sections, since it was observed that pigment bodies in the glial cells were more often clustered at one pole than were those in the neuron somata.

There is considerable lack of agreement among various investigators regarding the identification of glial types at the ultrastructural level (Kruger and Maxwell, 1966; Mori and Leblond, 1969a: King, 1968). However, on the basis of some recent studies (Mori and Leblond, 1969a, b) it seems probable that microglia and oligodendrocytes may be distinguished from astrocytes by the absence of glycogen granules, the absence of glio-fibrils, the presence of numerous free ribosomes and ribosomal rosettes, the presence of microtubules, and relatively dense nuclear chromatin masses. According to Mori and Leblond (1969a) microglia may be distinguished from oligodendroglia by the presence of smaller pleomorphic (usually elongated) nuclei, fewer microtubules and ribosomes, less rough endoplasmic reticulum (with cisterns often distended), fewer mitochondria, more extracellular spaces, and more dense bodies of various sizes. In our preparations we were unable to identify any features which were consistent enough to permit classifying the satellite glia as either oligodendrocytes or microglia, but on the basis of the structural characteristics described above, it appears that these cells cannot be classed as astrocytes.

The exact nature of the metabolic processes underlying the formation of lipofuscin pigment remains unknown although it is generally believed to result from the autoxidation and polymerization of unsaturated fatty substances in the cell. Regardless of the metabolic mechanisms underlying the formation of lipofuscin or whether the genesis of this pigment material is related to mitochondria (Hess, 1955), lysosomes (Samorajski, Ordy and Keefe, 1964/65), Golgi apparatus (Gatenby and Moussa, 1950; Gatenby, 1953) or other cell organelles, our present studies have demonstrated consistent differences in rate of accumulation and total amount of lipofuscin in cells of various strata of cerebral cortex.

In all cerebral cortical laminae the most consistent site of accumulation of the lipofuscin bodies is in the perikaryon just beneath the base of the apical dendrite. Samorajski, Ordy and Rady-Reimer (1968) have suggested that this characteristic distribution of the pigment "may have an important consequence for neuronal physiology". The data presented in the present report and in similar studies now in progress in our laboratories, should furnish a sound frame of reference to serve as a basis for future correlative studies of the possible relationship between lipofuscin accumulation and the physiologic characteristics and functional capabilities of neurons in both young and aged subjects.

References

Brizzee, K. R., Cancilla, P. A., Sherwood, N., Timiras, P. S.: The amount and distribution of pigments in neurons and glia of the cerebral cortex. Autofluorescent and ultrastructural studies. J. Geront. 24, 127—135 (1969).

Cammermeyer, J.: The postmortem origin and mechanism of neuronal hyperchromatosis and nuclear pyknosis. Exp. Neurol. 2, 379—405 (1960).

Chalkley, H. W.: Method for quantitative morphological analysis of tissues. J. Nat. Cancer Inst. 4, 47 (1943).

Einarson, L., Telford, I. R.: Structural changes in the nervous system of monkeys deprived of vitamin E. Anatomiske skrifter. 3, Nr. 1, Universitetsforlaget I Aarhus (1960a).

— — Effect of vitamin-E deficiency on the central nervous system in various laboratory animals. Biol. Skr. Dan. Vid. Selsk. 11(2), 1—81 (1960b).

Gatenby, J. B.: The golgi apparatus of the living sympathetic ganglion cells of the mouse, photographed by phase contrast. J. Roy. Micro. Soc. 73, 61—81 (1953).

— Moussa, T. A.: The sympathetic ganglion cell, with sudan black and the Zernike microscope, J. roy. micr. Soc. 70, 342—364 (1950).

Hess, A.: The fine structure of young and old spinal ganglia. Anat. Rec. 123, 339 (1955).

Karlsson, U., Schultz, R. L.: Fixation of the central nervous system for electron microscopy by aldehyde perfusion. I. Preservation with aldehyde perfusates versus direct perfusion with osmium tetroxide with special reference to membranes and the extracellular space. J. Ultrastruct. Res. 12, 160—186 (1965).

King, J. A.: A light and electron microscopic study of perineuronal glial cells and processes in the rabbit neocortex. Anat. Rec. 151, 111—124 (1968).

Krieg, W. J. S.: Connections of the cerebral cortex. I. The albino rat period A. Topography of the cortical areas. J. comp. Neurol. **84**, 221 (1946).

Kruger, L., Maxwell, D. S.: Electron microscopy of oligodendrocytes in normal rat cerebrum. Amer. J. Anat. **118**, 441—436 (1966).

Miyagishi, T., Takahata, N., Iizuka, R.: Electron microscopic studies on lipo-pigments in the cerebral cortex nerve cells of senile and vitamin E deficient rats. Acta neuropath. (Berl.) **9**, 7—17 (1967).

Mori, S., Leblond, C. P.: Identification of microglia in light and electron microscopy. J. comp. Neurol. **135**, 57—80 (1969a).

— — Electron microscopic features and proliferation of astrocytes in the corpus callosum of the rat. J. comp. Neurol. **137**, 197—226 (1969b).

Samorajski, T., Keefe, J. R., Ordy, J. M.: Intracellular localization of lipofuscin age pigments in the nervous system. J. Geront. **19**, 261—276 (1964).

— Ordy, J. M., Keefe, J. R.: The fine structure of lipofuscin age pigment in the nervous system of aged mice. J. Cell Biol. **26**, 779—795 (1965).

— — Rady-Reimer, P.: Lipofuscin pigment accumulation in the nervous system of aging mice. Anat. Rec. **160**, 555—574 (1968).

Schultz, R. L., Karlsson, U.: Fixation of the central nervous system for electron microscopy by aldehyde perfusion. II. Effect of osmolarity, pH of perfusate, and fixative concentration. J. Ultrastruct. Res. **12**, 187—206 (1965).

Sulkin, N. M.: In the process of aging in the nervous system (Edited by J. E. Birren, H. A. Imus and W. F. Windle). Springfield Ill.: Ch. C. Thomas 1959.

— Srivany, P.: Experimental production of senile pigments in nerve cells of young rats. J. Geront. **15**, 2 (1960).

THE EXPERIMENTAL PRODUCTION OF SENILE PIGMENTS IN THE NERVE CELLS OF YOUNG RATS*

NORMAN M. SULKIN, Ph.D. and PAKA SRIVANIJ, M.D., M.S.

Pigmentation of nerve cells is generally associated with senility; in fact the lipofuscin pigment is usually called senility pigment. Dolley and Guthrie (3) in reviewing the literature point to numerous early investigations and opinions concerning the role that pigmentation plays in aging.

Schäfer (13) presented the view that pigmentation can be interpreted as a sign of functional activity rather than decadence, since pigments were much more abundant in nerve cells of adults than in the nerve cells of children and lower animals. Hodge's (7) studies led him to conclude that pigmentation of nerve cells was related to senility. He observed that the cytoplasm of nerve cells from senile human individuals was largely filled with pigment, whereas the nerve cells of the fetus contained almost no pigment. White (24) concluded that the accumulation of pigment in the nerve cell of autonomic ganglia was due to loss of function. He showed that pigment in nerve cells decreased as the mammalian scale is descended until it is no longer observed. Therefore, he postulated that the autonomic ganglia become less and less im-

* This investigation was supported in part by Research Grant B-342, from the National Institute of Neurological Diseases and Blindness, Public Health Service.

67

portant as the animal scale is ascended until its minimum of importance is reached in man.

Dolley (2) observed that while pigment is associated with senility, it is because "in the duality of senility, i.e., senility of function and senility of depression, the factor of depression is almost inevitable in an organism."

A number of studies have been made on the characteristics and nature of the pigment in autonomic ganglion cells. Kuntz (9, 10) agreed with the majority of the early investigators as to the dual nature of the pigment. He found that the pigments in autonomic cells were of two kinds. One he identified as a yellow pigment, which reacts to fat stains and which is at least partially soluble in alcohol, ether, and other fat solvents. He described the other as a darker, more stable pigment, which did not react to fat stains and which was highly insoluble. This darker pigment was referred to as melanin. Spiegel and Adolf (15) further described this dark pigment (melanin) as arising from the yellow pigment. With advancing age, the yellow pigment commonly disappears, leaving only dark pigment in a majority of the autonomic ganglion cells. Truex (21) also concurred with the presence of melanotic pigment in autonomic nerve cells of persons of all ages.

Sympathetic ganglion cells containing both melanin and lipochrome pigments were described by Larsell (11). His work also supported the reports by Strong and Elwyn (16) that the lipochrome pigment was not present in nerve cells at birth but was found in increased amount with age.

Wolf and Pappenheimer (25) in their work on the nerve cell suggest that a chemical relationship exists between the pigment they described and the substance called ceroid reported by Lillie, Daft, and Sebrell (12) in their studies on livers of vitamin E-deficient rats. They also report that in their study of the dorsal sensory ganglia this pigment is present in addition to melanin but never in the same cell.

Sulkin (17) has further attempted to characterize the nature of pigment in autonomic nerve cells with the use of histochemical methods. He has observed pigmented ganglion cells in individuals ranging in age from 7 to 92 years. The data obtained as a result of his studies indicated that there were no melanotic pigments in human autonomic ganglion cells. No evidence was obtained, moreover, to support the view that lipid-containing pigments could be transformed into melanin. A comparison of pigment in autonomic ganglion cells and in human cirrhotic livers indicated that they have similar properties, which are both similar to the properties of ceroid. Later studies on the pigments of sensory ganglion cells, ventral horn cells, and Purkinje cells (18) showed similar results to those obtained with autonomic ganglion cells. D'Angelo, Issidorides, and Shanklin (1) studying the staining reactions of granules in the human neuron have confirmed these observations. On the basis of their findings, they agree with the writer that the pigment granules are similar to ceroid as well as to the vitamin E-deficient pigment.

There is no conclusive evidence to indicate whether pigmentation of nerve cells is due to an intrinsic factor of aging or whether the pigment is accumulated in the cell because of extrinsic environmental factors in which the factor of aging is coincidental. There is some support for the latter point of view. In experimental laboratory animals, where the environment is to some degree controlled, pigments do not accumulate in the nerve cell until the animal is senile. Even at this time, the deposition of pigment is not marked. In the dog, where the environment is controlled to a lesser degree, deposition of pigments in nerve cells again does not occur prior to old age. However, the accumulation of pigment in the senile dog is much greater than it is in the laboratory animal. In man, where the environment is even less controlled, the nerve cells are characterized by the presence of pigments in almost all age groups. The concentration of pigment varies markedly in different individuals irrespective of their age groups.

The present study has been designed to determine the possibility of producing pigments in the nerve cells of young rats by altering the environment so that data could be obtained concerning the role of extrinsic factors in the deposition of nerve cell pigments.

MATERIAL AND METHODS

The lipofuscin pigments in these experiments were visualized by the PAS technique following diastase digestion, which removed the glycogen. It has been demonstrated, however, that PAS positive mucoprotein granules occur in the cytoplasm of many neurons in various species (18, 19, 20). In order to distinguish the lipofuscin pigment from the mucoprotein granules, alternating sections were stained with Sudan black, oxidized with performic or peracetic acid prior to staining with the Schiff reagent, stained for acid fastness, and treated by the Schmorl (14) ferri-ferricyanide reduction test.

The following experiments were performed:

A. *Acetanilid experiments.*—Thirty-six young rats, 2 to 3 months of age, were given 3.7 mg./Kg. of acetanilid daily, by tubal administration for periods up to 90 days. At the end of 90 days, 18 of the animals were sacrificed, and the administration of acetanilid was discontinued in the remaining 18 rats. At the time of sacrifice of the animals, the brain, superior cervical ganglia, spinal ganglia, and spinal cord were removed, fixed in 10% formalin, dehydrated, embedded in paraffin, and sectioned in the routine manner. Successive sections from each tissue were treated with the PAS technique and with the other methods mentioned above.

The remaining 18 rats were placed on a diet of stock laboratory chow and were sacrificed at varying intervals in a period of from 6 months to 18 months following the cessation of the administration of the acetanilid.

B. *Hypoxic chamber experiments.*—Twenty young rats were placed in an anoxic chamber in which the amounts of oxygen and nitrogen that were introduced could be regulated. The oxygen level within the chamber was measured by means of an oxygen analyzer. The oxygen and nitrogen were controlled so that there was a gradual diminution of the former. From the fifth day to the twenty-first day the level of oxygen was maintained at from 5% to 8.9%.

70

The 8 animals which were still alive at the end of the 21st day were sacrificed, the nerve tissues were removed, fixed in formalin, and processed according to the manner described above.

C. *Vitamin E-deficiency experiments.*—One hundred and ten rats, from 6 weeks to 3 months of age, were placed on a vitamin E-deficient diet for periods up to 600 days. This diet had the following composition: 20% vitamin-free test casein GBI, 56% dextrose, 10% lard, 4% salt mixture (8), 10% brewer's yeast powder, together with the following fat-soluble vitamins per 100 pounds: 523 Gm. cod liver oil or 68 Gm. carotene in oil, GBI type 3a, and 0.001 Gm. calciferol. The rats were sacrificed at varying time intervals after being maintained on this diet 150 days or more and kept on a stock laboratory diet for 90 to 400 days before being sacrificed.

D. *ACTH experiments.*—Twenty-four rats, including 12 rats 4 months of age, 6 rats 8 months of age, and 6 rats 27 months of age, were separated into 3 groups. The first group served as controls. The second group underwent a unilateral nephrectomy. The third group was subjected to a unilateral nephrectomy, after which each animal received subcutaneous injection of 0.33 unit of ACTH gel per 100 Gm. of body weight every other day for 48 days beginning 10 days after the unilateral nephrectomy. The brains, spinal cords, autonomic ganglia, and sensory ganglia were dissected out, following fixation by perfusion, and were processed as described above.

The rats that were used in the acetanilid experiments and in the chronic anoxia experiments were of the Wistar (MW-2) strain. The vitamin E-deficiency experiments were performed on rats of the Wistar (MW-2), the C. F. Nelson, the HLA, the Long-Evans, and the Sherman strains. The rats which were subjected to unilateral nephrectomy and ACTH administration were of the C. F. Nelson strain.

RESULTS

A. *Acetanilid experiments.*—It is well known that the excessive or long continued use of cer-

71

tain nitrogen-containing compounds, particularly acetanilid, results in the formation of methemoglobin in the blood. This, in turn, could result in a condition of chronic anoxia.

It was noted that after three weeks of daily tubal administration of acetanilid the animals became extremely lethargic. Upon autopsy it was observed that all of the animals suffered from cranial subdural hemorrhages and clots. In some instances, subdural hemorrhages were noted in the spinal cord.

Examination of the blood showed a variation in the hematocrit from 32% to 54%, with a mean hematocrit of 48.5% as compared with an hematocrit of 39% in control animals. The hemoglobin (Haden-Hauser Scale) ranged from 10 to 13 Gm.% with a mean of 11.3 Gm.% as compared to a reading of 15.6 Gm.% in the control animals. Determination of methemoglobin by the microphotometric method of Evelyn and Malloy (6) in the experimental rats indicated a methemoglobin concentration of just below 50%.

In the group of animals which were sacrificed at intervals from 3 weeks to 40 days after the initiation of the experiment there was no indication of pigment deposition. The group which was sacrificed at varying intervals from 45 days to 90 days following the beginning of the experiment, on the other hand, was characterized by a deposition of lipofuscin in the cytoplasm of nerve cells from autonomic ganglia, sensory ganglia, ventral horn cells of the spinal cord, Purkinje cells, and from neurons in various areas of the brain (fig. 1). Control animals of the same age showed no indication of neuronal lipofuscin pigment.

In the remaining rats, which were sacrificed at various intervals in a period of 6 months to 18 months following the cessation of the administration of the drug, the lipofuscin pigment in the cytoplasm of the nerve cells occurred with a similar distribution and concentration as observed in the previous group (fig. 2).

In an ancillary experiment, 3 young dogs, including 1 dog 3 months old and 2 dogs approximately 6 months old, were given capsules con-

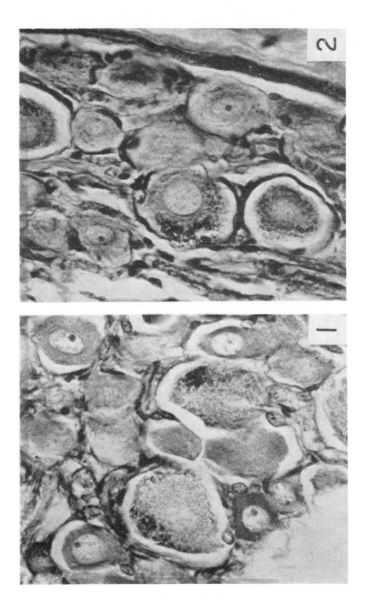

Fig. 1. Photomicrograph from section of spinal ganglion from young rat maintained on a daily supplement of acetanilid for 90 days, colored by the PAS reaction. 10X ocular, 48X objective.

Fig. 2. Photomicrograph from section of spinal ganglion from a rat which had been maintained on a stock diet for 8 months after cessation of the administration of acetanilid, colored by the PAS reaction. 10X ocular 48X objective.

taining, respectively, 24, 45, and 60 mg. of acetanilid daily for a period of 77 days. At the end of this period the nerve tissue which was removed, including specimens of all parts of the nervous system, was characterized by the presence of lipofuscin pigment in the cytoplasm of many of the nerve cells. In the normal, well-cared for dog, such pigment is usually not observed until the animal reaches an age of approximately 9 years.

B. *Hypoxic chamber experiment.*—Following the conditions described in the experiment, the animals that remained alive after 21 days were sacrificed and the various parts of the nervous system were dissected and processed. Numerous nerve cells from different parts of the nervous system of all of these animals were characterized by the presence of lipofuscin pigment in the cytoplasm (fig. 3).

C. *Vitamin E-deficiency experiments.*—In each instance in which the animals had been subjected to the vitamin E-deficient diet for 150 days or more, the cytoplasm of the nerve cells from various parts of the nervous system was characterized by large deposition of lipofuscin pigment (figs. 4, 5). The concentration of pigment was greater in the vitamin E-deficient animals than in the animals subjected to the other experimental procedures. Moreover, the concentration of this pigment was greater than is observed in the neurones of senile rats; even in rats which were only 210 days old at the termination of this experiment.

Some animals were removed from the vitamin E-deficient diet at various intervals after 150 days and were placed on the stock laboratory diet. In all such instances, the pigment was retained in the nerve cells even after intervals of more than 18 months (fig. 6).

D. *ACTH experiments.*—The control animals in the 4-month-old group of rats showed no indication of the deposition of lipofuscin pigments in nerve cells of any part of the nervous system which was examined. The rats of this age group which were examined 58 days following unilateral nephrectomy were characterized by the presence of small amounts of

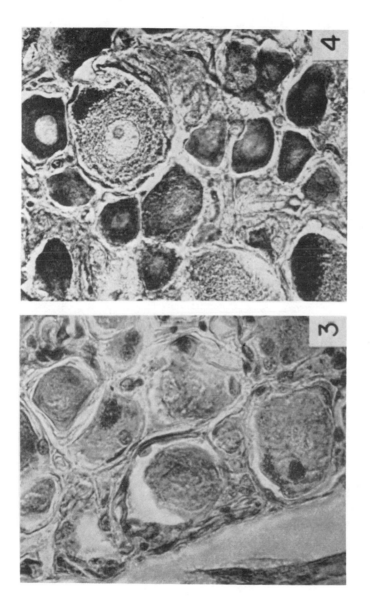

Fig. 3. Photomicrograph from section of spinal ganglion from young rat subjected to low oxygen tension for 21 days, stained with Sudan black. 10X ocular, 48X objective.

Fig. 4. Photomicrograph from section of spinal ganglion of rat maintained on a vitamin E-deficient diet for 245 days, stained with Sudan black. 10X ocular, 48X objective.

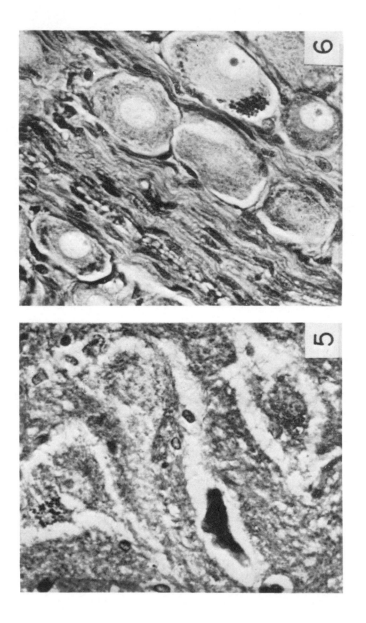

Fig. 5. Photomicrograph from section of spinal cord from young rat maintained on a vitamin E-deficient diet for 290 days, colored with the PAS reaction. 10X ocular, 48X objective.

Fig. 6. Photomicrograph from section of spinal ganglion of rat which had been maintained on a stock diet for 75 days after having been subjected to a vitamin E-deficient diet for 230 days, colored with the PAS reaction. 10X ocular, 48X objective.

lipofuscin pigment in the cytoplasm of a few scattered nerve cells in various portions of the nervous system. The ACTH-treated rats of this age group showed significant amounts of lipofuscin pigment in the cytoplasm of numerous nerve cells in all parts of the nervous system (figs. 7, 8).

In the normal rats of the 8-month-old group, occasional cells in various parts of the nervous system showed lipofuscin pigment in the cytoplasm. The rats of this age group which had been subjected to unilateral nephrectomy and to unilateral nephrectomy together with the administration of ACTH were similar in regard to the pigment distribution to the 4-month old groups which had undergone similar treatments.

The cytoplasm of numerous nerve cells in the 27-month-old series of normal rats contained depositions of lipofuscin pigment. This was particularly noticeable in autonomic ganglion cells, sensory ganglion cells, ventral horn cells, Purkinje cells, and cells of the pontine nuclei, although the pigments were also observed in other portions of the central nervous system. In relation to their pigment content, the nerve cells of the rats in this age group which had been subjected to unilateral nephrectomy could not be distinguished from the control group of senile animals. On the other hand, in the animals of this age group which had received ACTH, the cytoplasm of most of the nerve cells were characterized by large amounts of pigment. The amount of pigment was present in much greater concentration than is normally found in the nerve cells of senile rats and was comparable in amount to that which is present in nerve cells of vitamin E-deficient rats.

The latter group of experiments as well as the preceding experiment indicated that the sex of the animal did not seem to be concerned in the process of pigment deposition.

DISCUSSION

The data obtained in this study present evidence which supports the view that the production of lipofuscin pigments in nerve cells may be brought about by extrinsic factors, such

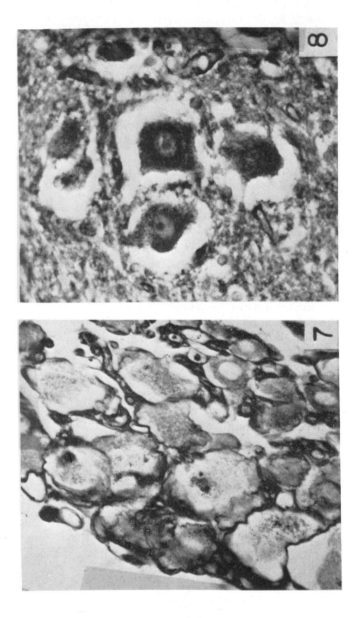

Fig. 7. Photomicrograph from section of spinal ganglion from 4-month-old female rat treated with ACTH for 48 days following unilateral nephrectomy, colored with the PAS reaction. 10X ocular, 48X objective.

Fig. 8. Photomicrograph from section of spinal cord from 4-month-old female rat treated with ACTH for 48 days following unilateral nephrectomy, colored with the PAS reaction. 10X ocular, 48X objective.

as environmental alterations, which are not related to the factor of aging. It further presents data which indicate that the production of pigment is a non-reversible phenomenon, that is, under the conditions of these experiments the pigment produced in nerve cells remains in the nerve cell indefinitely.

The determination of the production of chronic anoxia in the young animals by the administration of acetanilid was considered outside of the scope of the present studies. Although the deposition of pigment in the nerve cells resulted from such administration of the drug, it is not known whether this phenomenon was brought about by a lowering of the oxygen content, by a direct action of the acetanilid, the subdural hemorrhages, and their consequent effects, or as a result of other factors. The significance of this experiment was the demonstration that deposition of the so-called senile pigment could be initiated by experimentally altering the environment.

The occurrence or degree of anoxia, not having been determined in the above experiment, suggested the feasibility of constructing an anoxic cage which would enable us to have precise information concerning the oxygen environment of the animals. As has been demonstrated, the lowering of the oxygen level in the environment also resulted in the deposition of pigment in the nerve cells of young rats.

The deposition of lipoid products in the nervous system of vitamin E-deficient rats was first described by Einarson and Ringsted (4). Later, Einarson (5) further characterized this substance. The properties of this lipoidal substance are identical to the properties of the so-called senility pigment (17). Einarson's studies, as well as subsequent studies of other workers, were made on adult rats or without knowledge of the age of the animal. Since older rats are characterized by the presence of pigment in the nerve cells even in ordinary nutritive states, the present studies were performed on groups of rats which included very young animals. It has been demonstrated that a chronic vitamin E-deficiency, even in the youngest groups of animals, results in a deposition of lipofuscin pigment in the cytoplasm of the nerve cells. It is of further interest to note that vitamin E-deficiency results in a greater degree of pigmentation than is found following the other experimental procedures on the senile rats, even those between 1500 and 1600 days of age.

Wexler and Miller (22, 23) have suggested that excess pituitary-adrenal activity deserves further investigation as a possible mediator of the aging process and that exogenous ACTH may cause premature aging. Although it has been demonstrated in the present study that the administration of exogenous ACTH results in the deposition of senile pigments in the nerve cells of the young rat, there is no reason to believe that this procedure was responsible for the production of a premature aging. It is suggested, instead, that the deposition of the pigment was initiated by factors resulting from the stress associated with the increased ACTH rather than by a factor of premature aging. To support this view it is pointed out in these experiments that unilateral nephrectomy without ACTH administration apparently caused sufficient stress to produce pigments in the nerve cells of young rats and to increase the amount of pigment in in the nerve cells of older animals.

The data derived from these studies suggest the possibility that natural phenomena or alterations in the environment, including disease, nutritional deficiences, and emotional and physical stresses, could be considered as factors which initiate the deposition of lipofuscin pigments in nerve cells. It would not be unreasonable to assume that senile organisms are more susceptible to such factors. It is further suggested that the increased amount of pigment often observed in older individuals may represent an accumulation of such pigment during the life span.

SUMMARY

Thirty-six young rats, 2 to 3 months of age, when subjected to daily tubal administration of acetanilid for periods from 45 to 90 days are characterized by a deposition of lipofuscin pigments in the cytoplasm of their nerve cells. A discontinuance of the administration of the drug for periods of up to 18 months resulted in the continued presence of the pigment in the cytoplasm of these cells.

The occurrence of lipofuscin granules in the cytoplasm of nerve cells in 8 young rats was observed following the subjection of these animals to a lowered oxygen tension within an anoxic cage for a period of 15 days.

One hundred and ten young rats were maintained on a vitamin E-deficient diet for periods of 150 days to 600 days. Nerve cells in all of these rats were characterized by the presence of large amounts of lipofuscin pigment in the cytoplasm. Removal of the animals from this vitamin E-deficient diet for prolonged periods did not alter the occurrence and distribution of this pigment.

Twenty-four rats in different age groups, subjected to ACTH administration for a prolonged period of time following unilateral nephrectomy, were also characterized by either the occurrence or by an increase in the amount of lipofuscin pigment in the cytoplasm of the nerve cells.

It is suggested, as a result of the data obtained here, that senile pigmentation of nerve cells may be due to extrinsic factors rather than an aging factor.

REFERENCES

1. D'Angelo, C., Issidorides, M., and Shanklin, W.: A Comparative Study of the Staining Reactions of Granules in the Human Neuron, *J. Comp. Neurol.*, *106:* 487-499, 1956.

2. Dolley, D. H.: Studies on the Recuperation of Nerve Cells after Functional Activity from Youth to Senility, *J. Med. Res.*, *24:* 309-343, 1911.

3. Dolley, D. H., and Guthrie, F. V.: The Pigmentation of Nerve Cells. *J. Med., Res.*, *34:* 123-142, 1918.

4. Einarson, L., and Ringsted, A.: *Effect of Chronic Vitamin E Deficiency on the Nervous System and Skeletal Musculature in Adult Rats.* Levin and Munksgaard, Copenhagen, 1938.

5. Einarson, L.: Deposits of Fluorescent Acid-Fast Products in the Nervous System and Skeletal Muscles of Adult Rats with Chronic Vitamin-E-Deficiency, *J. Neurol., Neurosurg., & Psychiat.*, *16:* 98-109, 1953.

6. Evelyn, K. A., and Malloy, H. T.: Microdetermination of Oxyhemoglobin, Methemoglobin and Sulfhemoglobin in a Single Sample of Blood. *J. Biol. Chem., 126:* 655-662, 1938.

7. Hodge, C. F.: Changes in Ganglion Cells from Birth to Senile Death. Observations on Man and Honey-bee. *J. Physiol., 17:* 129-134, 1894.

8. Hubbel, R. B., Mendel, L. B. Wakeman, A. S.: A New Salt Mixture for Use in Experimental Diets, *J. Nutrition, 14:* 273-285, 1937.

9. Kuntz, A.: Sympathetic Ganglions Removed Surgically, A Histopathologic Study, *Arch. Surg., 28:* 920-135, 1934.

10. Kuntz, A.: Effects of Lesions of the Autonomic Ganglia, Associated with Age and Disease, on the Vascular System, *Biol. Symp. 11:* 101-117, 1945.

11. Larsell, O: *Anatomy of the Nervous System,* 2nd ed. Appleton-Century-Crofts, New York, 1950.

12. Lillie R. D., Daft, E. S., and Sebrell, W. H., Jr.: Cirrhosis of Liver in Rats on a Deficient Diet and the Effect of Alcohol, *Pub. Health Rep., 56:* 1255-1258, 1941.

13. Schäfer, E. A.: The Nerve Cell Considered as the Basis of Neurology, *Brain, 16:* 134-169, 1893.

14. Schmorl, G.: *Die pathologisch - histologischen Untersuchungsmethoden,* F. C. W. Vogel Leipzig, 1928.

15. Spiegel, A. E., and Adolf, M.: Die Ganglien des Grenzstranges, *Arb. neurol. Inst. Wien. Univ., 23:* 67-117, 1922.

16. Strong, O. S., and Elwyn, A.: *Human Neuroanatomy,* 2nd ed. Williams and Wilkins, Baltimore, 1948.

17. Sulkin, N. M.: Histochemical Studies of the Pigment in Human Autonomic Ganglion Cells, *J. Gerontol., 8:* 435-445, 1953.

18. Sulkin, N. M.: The Properties and Distribution of PAS Positive Substances in the Nervous System of the Senile Dog, *J. Gerontol., 10:* 135-144, 1955.

19. Sulkin, N. M.: Histochemical Studies on Mucoproteins in Nerve Cells of the Dog. *J. Biophys. & Biochem. Cytol., 1:* 459-468, 1955.

20. Sulkin, N. M.: The Distribution of Mucopolysaccharides in the Cytoplasm of Vertebrate Nerve Cells. *J. Neurochem.* (in press).

21. Truex, R. C.: Morphological Alterations in the Gasserian Ganglion Cells and Their Association with Senescence in Man. *Am. J. Path., 16:* 255-268, 1940.

22. Wexler, B. C., and Miller, B. F.: Severe Arteriosclerosis and Other Diseases in the Rat Produced by Corticotropin, *Science, 127:* 590-591, 1958.

23. Wexler, B. C., and Miller, B. F.: Age as a Factor in ACTH-Induced Arteriosclerosis in the Rat. *J. Gerontol., 12:* 430-431, 1957.

24. White, W. H.: Further Observations on the Histology and Function of the Mammalian Sympathetic Ganglia. *J. Physiol., 10:* 341-357, 1889.

25. Wolf, A., and Pappenheimer, A. M.: Occurrence and Distribution of Acid-Fast Pigment in the Central Nervous System, *J. Neuropath. & Exper. Neurol., 4:* 402-406, 1945.

Composition and Metabolism

THE REALITY OF AGE DIFFERENCES
IN NERVOUS TISSUE*

W. ANDREW, M.D., Ph.D.

The choice of the nervous system and particularly the neurons for investigation on cellular age changes is motivated by the fact that the nerve cells, because they do not reproduce after fetal or very early postnatal life, have a life span practically equal to that of the organism; such long-lived cells may therefore be expected to show age changes.

Our earlier investigations on the brain of the mouse (1, 2, 4, 5) and on the human brain (3, 7) resulted in findings which were in agreement with those of the majority of other workers on a variety of animals: dog (8, 10), rat (13), guinea pig (15), ape (11), and man (11, 12, 14). These observations have been reviewed recently by the present author (6) and will not be described in detail here. We may emphasize, however, that many positive findings have been reported. While different groups of nerve cells show different degrees and even types of alteration, certain general changes, such as diminution of Nissl material or decrease in the intensity of its basophilia, loss of clarity of the nucleus, and degenerative alterations leading to loss of cells, are very widespread.

* Supported by a grant from the Josiah Macy, Jr. Foundation.
We are much indebted for aid in the making of the preparations to Dr. C. E. McCreight, Mr. J. B. Taylor, and Mr. W. S. Belmont. The absorption studies on stained sections were performed by Dr. J. E. Kirk.

As new methods are developed in any field, it often becomes desirable to re-examine that field and the results obtained by workers who could not have employed these methods. At a conference on Aging of the Nervous System sponsored by the National Institute of Neurological Diseases and Blindness at Bethesda, a review was made of some of the earlier work in the field, and reports of several very recent investigations were made. The two most prominent features of these recent studies were 1) methods of fixation different from the "classical" immersion one were used and 2) the results in relation to age differences were largely or entirely negative.

These reports naturally lead to the question as to whether, in some way, the age differences described earlier have been brought about by the very process of preparation. It would seem that, even if the differences in the histological picture were thus brought about, some underlying difference of the nervous tissues of young and old animals in their reaction to the fixation process would have had to be present in the *fresh* tissue. Indeed, Gellerstedt (9), who studied an extensive series of human brains and described the presence of age differences, was inclined to ascribe the hypochromatism seen in large numbers of nerve cells in the senile brain to the occurrence of "preagonal changes" in the old brains due to a greater "vulnerability of their cells."

The points of view expressed at the Bethesda conference make necessary some re-examination of the age differences in the nervous system. It raises at least two important questions: 1) could the differences earlier described on material fixed by immersion have been due to some difference in "susceptibility" of cells at different ages and not to differences existing in living or in fresh tissue? and 2) if not, could most or all of these differences have been the result of errors of subjective interpretation by the investigators, due perhaps to an expectation and even a desire to see differences? The second possibility would be understandable perhaps on the basis of the subtle nature of some

87

of the differences described in populations of cells.

The present study was undertaken to investigate these problems. For this purpose we have studied nervous tissue of young and of senile animals, fixed by *perfusion* and we have reexamined the question of age differences seen in tissues fixed by immersion.

MATERIAL AND METHODS

The brains of 25 C57 Black mice have been studied. Three methods of preparation were used. The first involved fixation by perfusion. the second and third fixation by immersion.

The perfusion was carried out on 9 animals according to the directions of Windle (17). The ages of the mice included in the study are listed in table 1. After lightly anesthetizing the animal with ether, the thorax was opened, and a fine hypodermic needle (B-D Yale-lok 22G-1 1/4) was inserted into the left ventricle. Moderate pressure was used and the solutions flowed freely. The vascular system was then flushed with Solution A, approximately 10 cc. being used. The actual perfusion was then carried out with the same amount of Solution B. The inferior vena cava was opened to allow drainage of blood at the time of starting the flushing.

The cranial case was then opened, the brain was removed entire and stored in 10% formalin.

The compositions of Solutions A and B are as follows:

```
Solution A (for flushing)
    NaCl            9.0 Gm.
    Gum acacia     24.0 Gm.
    Formalin        2.0 cc.
    Distilled water      To make 1.0 L.
Solution B (for perfusion)
    NaCl            9.0 Gm.
    Gum acacia     24.0 Gm.
    Formalin      100.0 cc.
    Distilled water      To make 1.0 L.
```

Before dehydration the specimens were washed for two hours in running water. They were then passed through 30, 50, 70, 80, and 95% alcohol and two changes of absolute alcohol, remaining one hour in each solution. Two changes of xylol, each of 10 minutes' duration, followed, then two baths of warm paraffin of two hours each, and finally a third bath of overnight duration. The brains were embedded in histowax and sectioned at 10 μ.

For the staining procedure the sections were deparaffinized, hydrated, and stained for two min. in a 1% aqueous solution of cresyl violet. They were then washed in two changes of distilled water. Differentiation was begun in 95% alcohol, two min., continued for two min. in absolute alcohol, and completed in absolute alcohol to which had been added a trace of 10% colophonium in absolute alcohol (20 drops per 250 cc.). The final differentiation required 30 min. Clearing was carried out in 4 changes of xylol, 5 min. each, and the sections were mounted in Permount.

Six mice were used for preparation of the brains by ordinary immersion fixation with the other technical procedures exactly as for the perfused animals (immersion, method A, in table 1).

In addition to the mice thus used, nervous tissue from 10 other mice was prepared by immersion fixation and a somewhat different procedure in the other technical steps (immersion, method B, table 1). For the brains of these animals, fixation was in 10% formalin, where the tissue remained for from two hours to several days. They were then carried through 70,

TABLE 1. ANIMALS AND METHOD OF FIXATION.

Perfusion (Age in Days)	Immersion	
	Method A (Age in Days)	Method B (Age in Days)
83	37	128
179	59	129
208	169	129
209	192	130
608	629	134
613	659	497
622	...	555
668	...	590
809	...	596
...	...	597

80, 95, and 100% alcohol, remaining for periods of one-half to one hour in each. There followed alcohol-chloroform, one part chloroform with two of alcohol, then equal mixtures of alcohol and chloroform, then three parts chloroform to one of chloroform, and finally pure chloroform. The tissues remained in each of the fluids for from one hour to overnight. They were then placed in warm paraffin until the chloroform was removed, as determined by loss of odor, a time which was at most one hour. They were embedded in paraffin and sectioned, as were the tissues previously described. For staining, deparaffinization was carried out in xylol. After hydration, the sections were stained in 1% aqueous solution of cresyl violet for two min., washed in distilled water, differentiated as above in 95 and then 100% alcohol with final differentiation in absolute alcohol with colophonium as above, cleared, and mounted. Immersion fixation, method B, was used for comparison with the perfusion fixation and with immersion fixation, method A, because method B had been employed in preparing nervous tissue from a large number of specimens on which counts of binucleate cells were planned.

It is not easy to judge the relative value of one technical procedure as compared to another. Of the two methods of preparation employed for our material fixed by immersion, the one in which xylol rather than chloroform was employed in clearing before infiltration (method A) seemed somewhat preferable, as judged by a lesser amount of shrinkage of cell bodies and a smaller number of vacuoles in the interstitial material. The perfused material gave an appearance of very good fixation in all instances, if lack of pericellular spaces and of extracellular vacuoles are good criteria, and seemed somewhat superior to its counterpart, immersion, method A.

RESULTS

Two types of comparison of the brains of animals of different ages were made. In a gross comparison of the tissue samples a diffusely deeper stain of the brains of younger animals

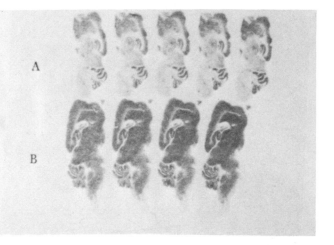

Fig. 1. *A*. Sagittal section of the brain of a 590-day-old C57 Black mouse. Immersion fixation, method B. X6.5. *B*. Sagittal sections of the brain of a 129-day-old C57 Black mouse. (A and B stained synchronously on same slide). Immersion fixation, method B. X6.5.

was observed. This was first noted on sections which had been mounted on separate slides but carried through the deparaffinization, hydration, staining, dehydration, and clearing processes together. It was confirmed by mounting sections of the brains of young and old animals on the same slides, in alternate rows. Figure 1 shows the magnitude of the age difference seen in material fixed by immersion, method B. The material fixed by perfusion showed a difference of lesser degree but similar type.

A study of the material for the light absorption characteristics of the standard sections, using a Beckman spectrophotometer, revealed a definite difference between the sections from the young and old mice. The absorption curve of the cresyl violet solution used in staining was of interest in showing a maximum located between the maxima for the stained tissue slides from the young and old animals.

The second type of comparison is that of the individual cells in the various regions of the brain. Since these have been described at

91

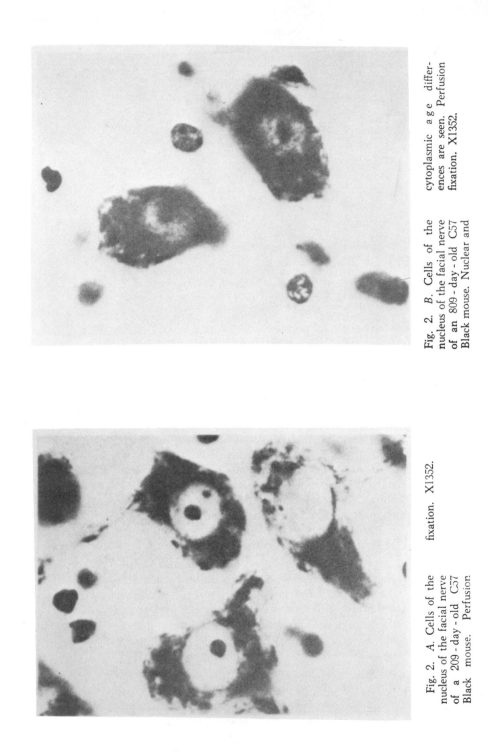

Fig. 2. *B*. Cells of the nucleus of the facial nerve of an 809 - day - old C57 Black mouse. Nuclear and cytoplasmic a g e differences are seen. Perfusion fixation. X1352.

Fig. 2. *A*. Cells of the nucleus of the facial nerve of a 209 - day - old C57 Black mouse. Perfusion fixation. X1352.

length previously for immersion-fixed material and recently reviewed (6), we may concentrate our description on the material fixed by perfusion. It is particularly on such material that negative results in relation to age change have been reported (16).

In our own perfusion-fixed material there seems to be a minimum of possible artifactual change, such as shrinkage or formation of extracellular or intracellular vacuoles. For the comparison of cell types in young and old animals we chose the Purkinje cells, the large motor cells of the nucleus of the facial nerve, and the cells of the dentate nucleus of the cerebellum.

The majority of Purkinje cells in the perfused brains from young animals show a content of abundant, discrete, and deeply stained granules of Nissl material. In such cells the nuclei generally are clear, sometimes sharply so, and the chromatin in relation to the nucleolus is very deeply stained (fig. 3-A). There always are some cells present in which, in contrast, the cytoplasm is deeply and almost homogeneously stained and in which the nuclei are obscured. Such cells are the so-called "chromophilic" cells.

In the perfused cerebella of the old animals the Purkinje cells show generally a rather lightly staining cytoplasm with few Nissl granules and those which are visible are more weakly staining (fig. 3-B). Chromophilic cells are present here also but do not stain as intensely as in the younger mice.

The Purkinje cells of senile animals show a number of aberrations of the nucleus. Among the more common of these are an eccentric position of the nucleolus (fig. 3-C) and a lobed condition of the nucleus, often suggesting a process of amitotic division (fig. 3-D).

While all of these age differences have been described previously, it is interesting to note that they are demonstrable in sections of brains fixed by perfusion and mounted and stained on the same slide.

The cells of the facial nucleus in the young animals are typical large motor cells. They contain large, discrete, heavily stained blocks of

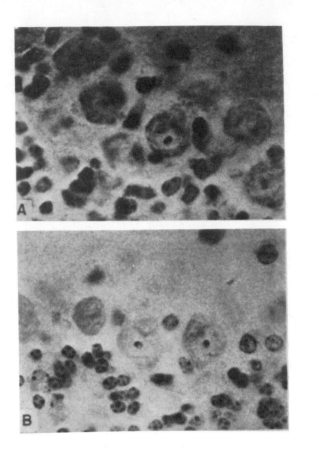

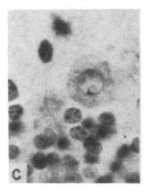

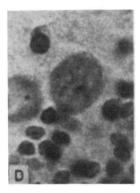

Fig. 3. *A*. Purkinje cells of the cerebellum of a 209-day-old C57 Black mouse. Nissl material is fairly abundant. *B*. Purkinje cells of the cerebellum of an 809-day-old C57 Black mouse. Nissl material is scanty. *C*. Eccentric nucleolus in Purkinje cell of an 809-day-old mouse. *D*. Aberrant form of nucleus in Purkinje cell of an 809-day-old mouse.

All cells in Figure 3 are from sections of brain fixed by perfusion and mounted and stained on the same slide. Cresyl violet. X1352.

Nissl substance (fig. 2A). The nuclei are very clear and the nucleoli sharply outlined with deeply stained chromatin granules. The cells of this nucleus in the senile mice present a considerably more varied appearance than in the young. Those chosen for illustration in figure 2B were selected as resembling most closely those in younger animals. They do show large blocks of Nissl material but there seems to be at least some qualitative age difference between the appearance of the cytoplasm, while the nuclei are considerably different, with powdery chromatin and less sharply defined nucleoli. There are individual cells and groups of cells in the facial nucleus of the old animals which are properly called hypochromatic, with very little Nissl material and often showing the nucleus and cytoplasm so similarly stained as to make differentiation between them very difficult.

The cells of the dentate nucleus in the perfused brains of young mice have discrete and deeply stained granules of Nissl material. The nuclei in many of the cells are clear and the nucleoli well defined with prominent chromatin associated with them. In the senile animals the majority of the cells are markedly different, with pale cytoplasm and scanty Nissl material. The nuclei show the powdery chromatin and the less regular appearance of the nucleoli seen in other areas in the old animals.

DISCUSSION

The result of this comparison of age differences as seen after fixation by the perfusion and immersion methods consists essentially in the affirmation that such age differences are seen with either type of fixation. They are of the same general type in perfused as in immersed tissues. The concept of the distinction between the nerve cells of young and old animals as "real" differences thus gains considerable ground. It is hoped that this concept may be still further tested in the future by comparisons of animals of different age groups in which fresh and even living cells can be employed.

It is important in this type of study to emphasize that we must not transfer conclusions too rapidly from one species to another. Our own positive results with perfused material from the mouse may contrast with negative results by others on the guinea pig due to a species difference rather than to differences in technical processes or interpretative ability.

SUMMARY

Twenty-five mice of the C57 Black stock have been studied in an attempt to see whether age differences, previously described, are affected by manner of fixation, in particular whether fixation by perfusion gives preparations in which such differences are less readily seen than in those made after fixation by immersion.

Synchronous staining of the sections of brain, e.g., staining of the sections from young and old mounted in alternate rows on the same slide, shows that brain tissue from young adults stains more deeply with cresyl violet than does that from old animals.

Individual cells, including the Purkinje cells and those of the facial nucleus and the dentate nucleus, show consistent age differences when perfused material is studied. These differences are similar to those seen in material fixed by immersion.

REFERENCES

1. Andrew, W.: The Nissl Substance of the Purkinje Cell in the Mouse and Rat from Birth to Senility. *Ztschr. f. Zellforsch. u. mikr. Anat., 25:* 583-604, 1936.

2. Andrew, W.: The Effects of Fatigue Due to Muscular Exercise on the Purkinje Cells of the Mouse, with Special Reference to the Factor of Age. *Ztschr. f. Zellforsch. u. mikr. Anat., 27:* 534-554, 1937.

3. Andrew, W.: The Purkinje Cell in Man from Birth to Senility. *Ztschr. f. Zellforsch. u. mikr. Anat., 28:* 292-304, 1938.

4. Andrew, W.: The Golgi Apparatus in the Nerve Cells of the Mouse from Youth to Senility. *Am. J. Anat., 64:* 351-375, 1939.

5. Andrew, W.: Neuronophagia in the Brain of the Mouse as a Result of Inanition and in the Normal Aging Process. *J. Comp. Neurol., 70:* 413-435, 1939.

6. Andrew, W.: Structural Alterations with Aging in the Nervous System. *Proc. Assn. Res. Nerv. & Ment. Dis., XXXV:* 129-170, 1956.

7. Andrew, W., and Cardwell, E. S., Jr.: Neurono-phagia in the Human Cerebral Cortex in Senility and in Pathologic Conditions. *Arch. Path., 29:* 400-414, 1940.

8. Dolley, D. H.: Further Verification of Functional Size Changes in Nerve Cell Bodies by the Use of the Polar Planimeter. *J. Comp. Neurol., 27:* 299-324, 1917.

9. Gellerstedt, N.: Zur Kenntnis der Hirnveränderungen bei der normalen Altersinvolution. *Upsala läkaref. förh., 38:* 193-408, 1933.

10. Harms, J. W.: Morphologische und experimentelle Untersuchungen an alternden Hunden. *Ztschr. Anat., 71:* 319-382, 1924.

11. Harms, J. W.: Alterserscheinungen im Hirn von Affen und Menschen. *Zool. Anz., 74:* 249-256, 1927.

12. Hodge, C. F.: Changes in Ganglion Cells from Birth to Senile Death. Observations on Man and Honeybee. *J. Physiol., 17:* 129-134, 1894.

13. Inukai, I.: Loss of Purkinje Cells with Age in the Albino Rat. *J. Comp. Neurol., 45:* 1-33, 1928.

14. Salimbeny, A. T., and Gery, I.: Contribution a l'Étude de l'Anatomie Pathologique de la Vieillesse. *Ann. Inst. Pasteur, 8:* 557-610, 1912.

15. Speigel, A.: Über die degenerativen Veränderungen in der Kleinhirnrinde im Verlauf des Individual-cyclus vom Cavia cobaya Marcgr. *Zool. Anz., 79:* 173-183, 1928.

16. Wilcox, H. H.: Changes accompanying Aging in the Brains of Guinea Pigs (Abstract). *J. Gerontol., 6 (Suppl. to No. 3):* 168, 1951.

17. Windle, W. F.: Personal Communication, 1957.

The Effects of Age on the Activity of Glutamic Acid Decarboxylase in Various Regions of the Brains of Rats

Melvin H. Epstein, MD, and Charles H. Barrows, Jr., ScD

AGE-DEPENDENT losses in skeletal muscle, a tissue composed of fixed postmitotic cells, were greater than those observed in liver, a tissue whose cells retain high regenerative capacity (Yiengst, Barrows, & Shock, 1959). It was proposed that enzyme systems which control the specialized functions of fixed postmitotic cells would most likely demonstrate age-associated changes (Barrows, 1966). Although brain has large populations of fixed postmitotic cells, i.e., neurons, it has been difficult to find many significant weight loss or biochemical differences of this tissue in old animals. Hollander and Barrows (1968) found no changes associated with senescence when calculated on the basis of DNA in the activities of enzymes which control nerve impulse transmission, viz, sodium-potassium activated adenosine triphosphatase or acetyl cholinesterase. Recently data have indicated that the glutamic acid decarboxylase (GAD) may also play an important role in the function and metabolism of neurons. For example, the studies of Bazemore (1956) and Florey (1954) suggest that gamma-aminobutyric acid (GABA), the product of the reaction catalyzed by GAD, is an inhibitory transmitter. In addition, a major biochemical shunt has been proposed which associates GAD with the tricarboxylic acid cycle. α-ketoglutaric acid is reductively aminated to glutamate which is decarboxylated by GAD to GABA. The GABA formed is converted to succinate semialdehyde which is oxidized to succinic acid (Bessman, Rossen, & Layne, 1953). This pathway is capable of diverting between 10-50% of the tricarboxylic acid substrates in brain tissue, (Machiyama, Baláz, & Julian, 1965; McKhann, Albers, Sokoloff, Michelsen, & Tower, 1960).

In this investigation the activities of GAD of prosencephalon, cerebellum, and brain stem of 2-, 12-, and 26-mo.-old rats were measured. The areas of the brains were also weighed to determine age associated changes in brain mass. In addition, studies were performed to compare the manometric measurement of GAD (Roberts & Frankel, 1951) with the $C^{14}O_2$ trapping procedure (Albers & Brady, 1959).

Materials and Methods

Animals.—Unmated female Wistar rats were used in this study. The animals were bred and maintained at the Gerontology Research Center (Baltimore). After weaning they were maintained four in a cage (25 cm. x 40 cm. x 17.5 cm.) at 21-22 C. and 50-55% relative humidity. They were offered Ralston Purina Laboratory Chow and water *ad libitum.* Ten animals were used in each of three groups with mean ages of 2 mo. ± 3 days, 12 mo. ± 4 days, and 26 mo. ± 6 days. Two 15-mo.-old animals were used to confirm the manometric technique by $C^{14}O_2$ trapping.

Tissue preparations.—All animals were decapitated and the brains rapidly removed and chilled. The time interval from decapitation to placement in crushed ice never exceeded 60 sec. The prosencephalon was then removed rostral to a transverse incision at Craigie's level A9 (Zeman & Innes, 1963). Superiorly the sectioning began just posterior to the corpus pineale, and subsequently passed through the colliculus posterior, nucleus tegmenti dorsalis, and nucleus tegmenti ventralis. The olfactory lobes were included in the prosencephalon sample. The cerebellum included all tissue superior to the inferior, middle and superior cerebellar peduncle. The remaining brain extending caudal to the pyramidal decussation was taken as brain stem.

The wet weights of the individual brain regions were then determined to the nearest milligram on an Ainsworth Type S precision balance. Homogenates (37.5%) were prepared using distilled water with a teflon pestle in a glass homogenizer tube immersed in crushed ice.

Enzymatic Assays

Manometric—Glutamic acid decarboxylase activity was measured by the Warburg manometric method at 37.0 C. as the microliters of CO_2 released per hour (Roberts & Frankel, 1951). The final volume of substrate-buffer in each flask was 3.4 cc. and contained 2.0×10^{-2}M glutamic acid pH 6.4, 1.0×10^{-2}M malonic acid pH 6.4, 4.0×10^{-4}M pyridoxal phosphate and $0.1 M \times 10^{-2}$ sodium phosphate buffer pH 6.4. All flasks were gassed for 10 min. with pre-purified nitrogen, equilibrated for 10 min., then combined with 150 mg. of homogenated brain from the side arm. Readings were taken every 10 min. for 60 min.

$C^{14}O_2$ *trapping.*—The incubation medium was placed in the bottom of a 10 cc. glass injectable container (Weaton Co.) with a 0.75 ml. pyrex cup suspended from a platinum wire inserted through the rubber stopper. The stopper was then secured to the bottle using an aluminum cap with a matched capper. After gassing for 10 min. with pre-purified nitrogen using two 20 gauge needles, 150 mg. of brain homogenate obtained from 15-mo.-old animals was injected into the reaction mixture through the rubber stopper. The incubation medium contained 2.0×10^{-2}M glutamic $-1 -C^{14}$ acid (sp. act. 5.18×10^{-3} μc/mM, pH 6.4, New England Nuclear), 1.0×10^{-2} M malonic acid (pH 6.4), 4.0×10^{-4}M pyridoxal phosphate, and 0.1 M sodium phosphate buffer pH 6.4. All flasks were shaken continuously in an Aminco water bath at 37.0 C. Twenty minutes before the termination of the reaction 0.5 cc. of the hydroxide of hyamine $10 - X$ (Rohm & Hass,

Inc.) was injected through the rubber stopper into the small suspended cup in the reaction chamber. The 0.5 cc. of hyamine was transferred quantitatively into 14.0 cc. of counting fluid which consisted of 4.0 gm/liter, 2,5 diphenyloxazole, and 0.05 gm/liter 1,4-bis 2-(5-phenyloxazolyl)-benzene in toluene. Counts were made in the Packard Tri-Carb Model 3375.

RESULTS

Total and regional brain weights were found to increase significantly ($p = 0.05$-0.001) with increasing age (Table 1). The exceptions were the prosencephalon between 2 and 12 mo. and 12 and 26 mo.

The glutamic acid decarboxylase activity per mg. of tissue did not show a statistical difference between 2-, 12-, and 26-mo.-old animals for the three brain regions studied (Table 2).

Marked significant differences ($p = 0.01$-0.001) in GAD activity were found between all brain regions within individual age groups except between the cerebellum and brain stem at 2 mo. (Table 2).

Table 1. The Effect of Age on the Weights of Various Regions of the Brains of Female Rats.

Age (Mo.)	2	12	26
N	10	10	10
Brain Stem	272+22[a]	359±19	460±14
Cerebellum	219±7	261±10	300±15
Prosencephlon	1,108±31	1,182±19	1,192±18
Total	1,599±42	1,802±22	1,952±24

[a]Mg Wet Weight, Mean ±SE_M.

Table 2. The Effect of Age on the Concentration of Glutamic Acid Decarboxylase in Various Regions of the Brains of Female Rats.

Age	2 Mo.	12 Mo.	24 Mo.
N	10	10	10
Brain Stem	266.0±29.9[a]	264.8±14.0	264.0±16.6
Cerebellum	338.1±24.0	350.2±19.3	321.6±12.7
Prosencephalon	423.1±17.9	441.9±17.3	425.0±12.0

[a]μl CO_2/hr/gm Wet Weight, Mean ±SE_M.

Total GAD activity (Table 3) was found to increase significantly in the cerebellum between all age groups (2-12 mo. $p = 0.042$, 12-26 mo. $p = 0.004$). In the brain stem there was a significant increase only between 2 mo. and 26 mo. ($p = 0.016$). No significant changes were found in the prosencephalon.

The activity of GAD in 150 mg. of two different brain homogenates was 60.0 μl CO_2/hr. and 61.0 μl. CO_2/hr. by the Warburg technique and 57.6 μl CO_2/hr. and 59.0 μl CO_2/hr., respectively, by the trapping technique. These data confirm the validity of the GAD activity measured by the manometric technique.

Table 3. The Effect of Age on the Total Activity of Glutamic Acid Decarboxylase of Various Regions of the Brain of Female Rats.

Age	2 Mo.	12 Mo.	24 Mo.
N	10	10	10
Brain Stem	77±11[a]	98±7	119±11
Cerebellum	53±3	71±5	97±6
Prosencephalon	479±27	537±19	507±16

[a] μl CO_2/hr/brain region, Mean ± SE_M.

DISCUSSION

The significant increase in brain weight during the first 12 mo. of life is in agreement with the findings of Hollander and Barrows (1968). In addition both the studies of Brizzee, Sherwood, and Maras (1968) and Neumaster and Ring (1955) demonstrated larger brains in 25- to 32-mo.-old animals than in 4- to 7-mo.-old rats. In the former study only the ratio of brain weight to body weight and the body weight of the animals were presented so that statistical analyses of the increments were not possible. Therefore, increases in brain mass appear to occur during growth and even young adult life.

Data presently available are not in agreement as to the effect of senescence on brain mass. In contrast to the present study, Hollander and Barrows (1968) found no significant changes in the weights of the brains of 10- to 12- and 26- to 32-mo. old rats. On the other hand, Smith (1930) reported that the brain weights of 1-, 2-, and 3-year-old animals were 2024 ± 28.5, 1977 ± 24.6 and 1911 ± 40, respectively. Although statistically significant age decrements were observed during the last 2 years of life, the magnitude of this change was only 5%, and the level of significance may be considered minimal ($p = 0.05$). Therefore, these data indicate that senescence does not result in a marked loss of brain tissue in rodents. Since the brain contains other cells in addition to neurons, it is possible that neural loss is accompanied by a glial or fibroblast proliferation so that total brain weight is unaffected by senescence. However, the lack of a decrease in the activity of GAD, expressed as the total activity or activity per unit wet weight of brain, suggests that the neurons are not lost during aging. This conclusion is supported by the data of Brizzee et al. (1968) that demonstrated a constant number of neurons per unit volume of cerebral cortex in 4-mo.-old and 24- to 32-mo.-old rats. It should be understood, however, that the concentration of enzyme per synaptic ending, or the number of synaptic endings, could change with age. This would leave in doubt any conclusions regarding age-associated changes in neuronal populations.

It is generally accepted that neurons do not increase in number after maturation (Allen, 1912; Byams, 1959). Therefore the continued growth of the brain even into late life would suggest an increase in the number of glia cells, fibroblasts, or myelin with age. In support of the glial theory, Brizzee et al. (1968) reported a 50% increase in the numbers of astrocytes and oliodendroglia cells per volume of cerebral cortex of rats between 4- and 25- to 32-mo.-old rats. In addition, the increase in the total activity of GAD suggests an age-associated increment in the enzymatic activity of neurons. Since the enzyme appears to be located in the synaptic vesicles (Balázs, Dahl, & Harwood, 1966; Salganicoff & De Robertis, 1963; Shatunova & Sytinsky, 1964; Van Kemper, Van Den Berg, Van Der Helm, & Veldstra, 1965; Weinstein, Roberts, & Kakefuda, 1963), an age-associated increase in the number of activities of GAD in these vesicles may be inferred. Finally the lack of an effect of age per unit wet weight of tissue suggest that these changes occur at essentially the same rate.

SUMMARY

Wet weights and the glutamic acid decarboxylase activities were determined in the prosencephalon, brain stem, and cerebellum of 2-, 12-, and 26-mo.-old female rats.

Total and regional brain weights were found to increase significantly with increasing age. The exceptions were the prosencephalon between 2 mo. and 12 mo. and 12 mo. and 26 mo.

The glutamic acid decarboxylase activity per mg. of wet tissue did not change with age in the three brain regions studied.

The total activity of glutamic acid decarboxylase increased significantly in the cerebellum between all age groups; and in the brain stem only between 2 mo. and 26 mo. No significant changes were found in the prosencephalon.

REFERENCES

Albers, R. N., & Brady, R. O. The distribution of GAD in the nervous system of the rhesus monkey. *Journal of Biological Chemistry,* 1959 **234**, 926-928.

Allen, E. The creation of mitosis in the central nervous system of the albino rat. *Journal of Comparative Neurology,* 1912, **22**, 547-568.

Balázs, R., Dahl, S., & Harwood, J. R. Subcellular distribution of enzymes of glutamate metabolism in rat brain. *Journal of Neurochemistry,* 1966, **13**, 897-905.

Barrows, C. H., Jr. Enzymes in the study of biological aging. In N. W. Shock (Ed.), *Perspectives in experimental gerontology.* Springfield, Ill.: Charles C Thomas, 1966.

Bazemore, A., Elliott, K. A. C., & Florey, E. Factor I and GABA. *Nature,* 1956, **178**, 1052-1053.

Bessman, S. R., Rossen, J., & Layne, E. C. GABA transamination in brain. *Journal of Biological Chemistry,* 1953, **201**, 385-391.

Brizzee, K. R., Sherwood, N., & Maras, P. S. T. A comparison of cell populations at various depth levels in cerebral cortex of young adult and aged Long-Evans rats. *Journal of Gerontology,* 1968, **23**, 289-297.

Byams, W. A. Mitotic activity in the brain of the adult rat. *Anatomical Record,* 1959, **133**, 65-74.

104

Florey, E. Inhibitory and excitatory factor of mammalian central nervous system and their action on single sensory neurons. *Archives internationales de physiologie*, 1954, **62**, 33-53.

Hollander, J., & Barrows, C. H., Jr. Enzymatic studies in senescent rodent brains. *Journal of Gerontology*, 1968, **23**, 174-179.

Machiyama, Y., Balázs, R., & Julian, T. Oxidation of glucose through the GABA pathway in the brain. *Biochemical Journal*, 1965, **96**, 68-69.

McKhann, G. M., Albers, W. R., Sokoloff, L., Michelsen, O., & Tower, D. B. The quantitative significance of the gamma-amino butyric acid pathway in cerebral oxidative metabolism. In E. Roberts (Ed.), *Inhibition in the nervous system and gamma-amino butyric acid*. New York: Pergamon Press, 1960.

Neumaster, T. D., & Ring, G. C. Creatine excretion and its relation to whole body potassium and muscle mass in inbred rats. *Journal of Gerontology*, 1965, **20**, 379-382.

Roberts, E., & Frankel, S. Glutamic acid decarboxylase in brain. *Journal of Biological Chemistry*, 1951, **188**, 789-795.

Salganicoff, L., & De Robertis, E. Subcellular distribution of GAD and GAB alpha-ketoglutamic transaminase. *Life Sciences*, 1963, **2**, 85-91.

Shatunova, N. F., & Sytinsky, I. A. On the intracellular locations of GAD and GABA in mammalian brain. *Journal of Neurochemistry*, 1964, **11**, 701-708.

Smith, C. G. The specific gravity of the brain of the male albino rat. *Journal of Comparative Neurology*, 1930, **50**, 97-108.

Van Kempen, G. M. T., Van Den Berg, C. J., Van Der Helm, H. J., & Veldstra, H. Intracellular localization of glutamate decarboxylase, GABA-T and some other enzymes in brain tissue. *Journal of Neurochemistry*, 1965, **12**, 581-588.

Weinstein, H., Roberts, E., & Kakefuda, T. Studies of subcellular distribution of GABA and glutamate decarboxylase in mouse brain. *Biochemical Pharmacology*, 1963, **12**, 503-509.

Yiengst, M. J., Barrows, C. H., Jr., & Shock, N. W. Age changes in the chemical composition of muscle and liver in the rat. *Journal of Gerontology*, 1959, **14**, 400-404.

Zeman, W., & Innes, J. R. M. *Craigie's neuroanatomy of the rat*. New York: Academic Press, 1963.

INFLUENCE OF AGE ON MONOAMINE OXIDASE AND

CATECHOL-O-METHYLTRANSFERASE IN RAT TISSUES

Arthur J. Prange, Jr.,Janice E. White,Morris A. Lipton and A. Marcine Kinkead

University of North Carolina School of Medicine, Chapel Hill, North Carolina

(Received 16 November 1966; in final form 19 December 1966)

The metabolism of catecholamines, principally norepinephrine, is currently

the focus of interest in a variety of regulatory processes and disease states

involving the sympathetic and central nervous system. Interest in this area

is reflected in recent reviews of synthesis (1) and degradation of the catechol-

amines (2).

At least two major illnesses, depression and schizophrenia, are age-

related; the former peaking at physiological involution, the latter following

adolescence. Both illnesses have been claimed to involve alterations or

aberration in catecholamine metabolism, and the literature on these subjects

has been recently reviewed (3,4). Therefore, it was of interest to study

the metabolism of catecholamines as a function of age and sex. The following

report deals with monoamine oxidase (MAO) and catechol-o-methyltransferase

(COMT), the enzymes involved in the destruction of norepinephrine.

Materials and Methods

Sprague-Dawley rats were obtained from a single commercial source. Some

rats were killed shortly after arrival while others were housed and fed under

standard conditions until they had reached the desired ages. Sick or moribund

rats were discarded. Rats were killed by decapitation. The experiment was

carried out over two years. Some young rats were killed during the end of

this period; some old rats were killed during the middle. MAO was determined

in the left lobe of the liver, left half of the brain, and the tip of the ventricle of the heart; COMT was determined in the left lobe of the liver, left half of the brain, and the inferior pole of the left kidney. (MAO activity was found to be low in kidney; less than 20% liver values; COMT activity was low in heart: less than 2% liver values.)

Tissues were removed from freshly killed rats, weighed and homogenized in isotonic KCl. In the MAO assay ^{14}C-tryptamine was used as a substrate and the enzymatically formed ^{14}C-indoleacetic acid, extracted into toluene, was measured by scintillation counting (5). In the COMT assay homogenate was incubated with epinephrine and ^{14}-C-Sadenosylmethionine. ^{14}C-metanephrine was extracted into a mixture of toluene and isoamyl alcohol at pH 10 and measured by scintillation counting (6). All values for both enzymes were determined in duplicate.

Results

Values for both enzymes in both sexes in all tissues were plotted according to age. On inspection of these data it was found that in both sexes MAO and COMT activity in liver appeared to rise about the ninth week and to decline about the 35th. On the basis of this observation all determinations were grouped into three time spans, or epochs: 2-9 weeks (mean, 5); 9-35 weeks (mean, 24); 35-100 weeks (mean, 67). Nine weeks is the approximate time of onset of sexual fertility in the laboratory rat (7).

Six separate analyses of variance were performed, one for each tissue and enzyme. The scores were analyzed for the presence of three effects. The "epoch" effect asked if there were significant differences between the means of the early, middle and late epochs (disregarding sex). The "sex" effect asked if all males and all females differed. The "epoch by sex" interaction tested whether the results across epochs were essentially similar for males and females.

In both males and females both MAO ($p < .01$) and COMT ($p < .001$) activity in liver increased during the middle epoch (Fig. 1). In the case of MAO the

107

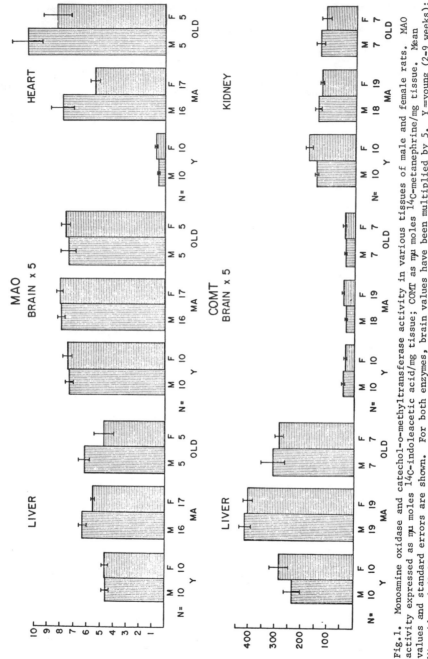

Fig.1. Monoamine oxidase and catechol-o-methyltransferase activity in various tissues of male and female rats. MAO activity expressed as mμ moles 14C-indoleacetic acid/mg tissue; COMT as mμ moles 14C-metanephrine/mg tissue. Mean values and standard errors are shown. For both enzymes, brain values have been multiplied by 5. Y =young (2-9 weeks); MA =mid-aged (9-35 weeks); OlD =35+ weeks.

increase was greater in males (p<.05). It can be seen that the mid-age enzyme activity increase in liver is relatively greater for COMT than for MAO.

In the brain the activity of both enzymes was constant throughout the life span of both sexes. Neither epoch, sex, nor interactive effects were found. It should be noted that brain has only about one third the MAO activity of liver; brain has only about one-sixtieth the COMT activity of liver.

MAO activity increased in the heart throughout the life span (p<.001). This was true for both sexes and there was no significant difference between the sexes. COMT activity in kidney decreased with age (p<.01) in both sexes, and there was no significant difference between sexes.

Discussion

Studer et al., using a histochemical technique, previously reported a marked increase in cardiac MAO in rats during the first 14 months of life (8). Male adult rats have been reported to have more MAO activity than females in both heart (9) and liver (10). These findings of other workers are corroborated here.

Testosterone elevates female hepatic MAO; estradiol lowers male hepatic MAO (11). After five weeks castration has no effect in either sex (11). This latter finding seems at odds with the present data, in which hepatic MAO activity declines in old rats. However, other influences than sexual involution may have been at work in our animals, some of which were very old. Apparently surgical castration and physiological aging may have quite different effects. Karki et al., have shown a marked increase in brain MAO from the newborn period to adult life (12). This finding is not incompatible with our data since our youngest rat was 15 days old.

Our data demonstrate that in mid-aged rats there is an increase in both COMT and MAO activity in liver. COMT increases more than MAO, suggesting that in this organ methylation rather than oxidative deamination may be the predominant pathway for amine degradation in young adult animals. This is offset,

109

however, by the findings of increasing MAO activity in heart and decreasing COMT activity in kidney. Because of the differences in size of these organs, differences in blood flow and substrate availability, allosteric effects and other factors, it is not possible to determine from these experiments the degree to which these alternate pathways are used in vivo. Wurtman and Axelrod (11), for example, have shown that cardiac MAO is present in considerable excess of utilization, since 50% inhibition has no effect upon the rate of disappearance of administered catecholamine. Nevertheless, the data are suggestive, since Blumberg and Klein (13) have noted a positive relationship in humans between increasing age and methoxy-catecholamine excretion.

It is apparent that definitive conclusions regarding the degree to which methylation and oxidative deamination are used for catecholamine degradation at different periods in life require experiments with the intact animal in vivo.

Summary and Conclusions

In mid-aged rats there is an increase in liver in both MAO and COMT activity, the COMT increase being relatively greater. MAO activity in heart increases with age; COMT activity in kidney decreases with age. The activity of both enzymes in brain is constant across all age groups.

Acknowledgements

We thank Dr. Carl M. Cochrane for his statistical help. This work was supported in part by USPHS grants 5-K3-MH-22536-05 and 5-K3-MH-18642-05.

References

1. Sidney Udenfriend, The Harvey Lectures, Series 60, 1964-65.

2. I.J. Kopin, in Actions of Hormones on Molecular Processes, G. Litwack, Ed. John Wiley & Sons, New York (1964), p. 257.

3. J.J. Schildkraut, Amer. J. Psychiat. 122, 509 (1965).

4. A.J. Friedhoff and E. Van Winkle, Amer. J. Psychiat. 122, 1054 (1965).

5. R.J. Wurtman and J. Axelrod, Biochem. Pharm. 12, 1439 (1963).

6. J. Axelrod, Personal communication.

7. William S. Spector, Ed., Handbook of Biological Data, W.B. Saunders (1956).

8. A. Studer, H.R. Baumgartner and K. Reber, Histochemie $\underline{4}$, 43 (1964).

9. R.G. Skillen, C.H. Thieves and L. Strain, Endocrinol. $\underline{70}$, 743 (1962).

10. R.J. Wurtman, I.J. Kopin and J. Axelrod, Endocrinol. $\underline{73}$, 63 (1963).

11. R.J. Wurtman and J. Axelrod, Biochem. Pharm. $\underline{12}$, 1417 (1963).

12. N. Karki, R. Kuntzman and B.B. Brodie, J. Neurochem. $\underline{9}$, 53 (1962).

13. A.G. Blumberg and D.F. Klein, J. Psychiat. Res. $\underline{3}$, 239 (1965).

Changes in Dephosphorylating Enzymes in Young and Old Tissues of the Rat

A preliminary communication

By GEOFFREY H. BOURNE

In view of the changes, both physiological and morphological which take place in older animals and since the systems of phosphorylation and dephosphorylation play an important part in energy exchanges in the living cell, it seems important to study the ability of various tissues from young and old animals to dephosphorylate various phosphate esters.

Material and Methods

6 male rats 3 months old and 6 male rats 3 years old were used for this work. They were killed by a blow on the neck. The tissues upon removal were fixed at once in chilled alcohol, embedded in wax and sectioned in the usual way. The following sixteen organs were studied – cerebrum, cerebellum, liver, heart, kidney, skeletal muscle, adrenal, seminal vesicles, testis, thyroid, trachea, pituitary, salivary glands, pancreas, skin and duodenum.

Phosphatase activity was detected by the standard Gömöri procedure. The incubation time for each tissue was varied according to the phosphatase activity of the organ. To ensure adequate comparison of activity slides of the same organs of young and old animals were incubated and carried through the various visualization procedures together.

The phosphate esters used (all with one exception pH 9.0) were glycerophosphate which presumably demonstrates what is colloquially called "alkaline phosphatase" which is in fact, a nonspecific phosphomonoesterase, oestrone- and cortisone-phosphates, pyridoxal-phosphate, carbamyl-phosphate and ethanolamine-phosphate. The enzymes which dephosporylate these latter compounds although having their optimum pH is in the region if 8–9 appear to be quite distinct from the non-specific "alkaline phosphatase". The histochemical preparations which are obtained from their use are quite different from those obtained from the latter.

112

Results

When the steroid- phosphates and also ethanolamine- and carbamyl-phosphates are used as substrates the reaction is predominantly in the nuclei, but there is a cytoplasmic reaction also, particularly in neurones, and it is greater in all cells of the organs of older animals. Pyridoxal-phosphate gives a stronger cytoplasmic than nuclear reaction, both are increased in old age – the same applies to the other substrates used. In this preliminary paper only the more outstanding results are recorded in detail, a fuller paper will be published in due course.

Cerebellum

When cortisone-phosphate is used as a substrate, the nuclei of the cells of the nuclear layer in the young animal give a very strong positive reaction, there is also a slight reaction in their cytoplasm and in the surrounding fibres. The molecular layer and the basket cell nuclei give a very strong reaction. The Purkinje cells, on the other hand show a slight reaction in both cytoplasm and nuclei although when the section passes through nucleolus it is much more positive than the rest of the nucleus. It is of interest that the "basket" fibres around the bodies of the Purkinje cells give quite a strong reaction (fig. 1).

In the older animal the Purkinje cells can be seen to be reduced in size and the cytoplasm gives a stronger reaction than in the control. A stronger positive reaction is given by an area on one side of the nucleus which appears to be the Golgi apparatus. The nuclei of the cells of the nuclear layer and the fibres of the molecular layer give a much stronger reaction. The "basket" fibres around the Purkinje cells were not as positive as in the control (fig. 2).

With pyridoxal-phosphate at an acid pH there was a moderate reaction in most parts of the cerebellum in the young animal and a stronger one in the old animal. The cytoplasm of the Purkinje cells in the latter was much more positive and a strong reaction was given by an area near the nucleus which was almost certainly the Golgi apparatus (figs. 3 and 4).

Brain Stem

Many of the neurones in the nuclei of the brain stem give a strong reaction with a variety of substrates. For the purposes of this

113

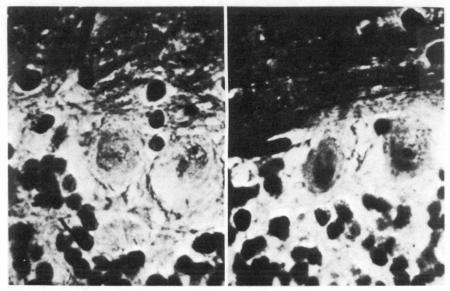

Fig. 1   Fig. 2

Fig. 1. Purkinje cells in young animal. *Substrate:* cortisone-phosphate.

Fig. 2. Purkinje cells in old animal. *Substrate:* cortisone-phosphate.

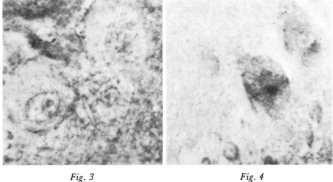

Fig. 3   Fig. 4

Fig. 3. Purkinje cells in young animal. *Substrate:* acid pyridoxal-phosphate.

Fig. 4. Purkinje cells in old animal. *Substrate:* acid pyridoxal-phosphate.

paper however we will refer only to the neurones from the region of the origin of the motor root of the 5ᵗʰ nerve and the substrate used was ethanolamine-phosphate at pH 9.0.

In the young animal a very strong reaction was given by the nucleolus and a moderate reaction by the chromatin of the nucleus and by the nuclear membrane. A slightly less intense reaction was given by the cytoplasm. A moderate reaction was also given by the surrounding fibres (fig. 5).

In the old animal the nucleus had become more vesicular the nucleolus larger and more reactive and the larger masses of chromatin also stained more deeply. The reaction was much less obvious in the nuclear membrane but was considerably increased in the cytoplasm and in the surrounding nerve fibres (fig. 6).

Pituitary

Oestrone-phosphate at pH 9.0 gave a reaction in the young animal almost exclusively in the nuclei and largely in the chromatin (fig. 7). In the older animal this nuclear reaction became restricted to the nucleoli and the nuclear membrane but showed up also in the cytoplasm and in the cytoplasmic membrane (fig. 8).

Adrenals

In the young animals the adrenals with pyridoxal-phosphate at pH 9.0 gave a general positive reaction in all the cortical cells, but this was slightly more intense in the three or four layers of the zona glomerulosa. The reaction was largely cytoplasmic – both diffuse and granular but there was also a positive reaction in the nucleoli and the nuclear membrane (fig. 9).

In old animals this positive zone was greatly increased – to about twelve layers of cells. The reaction in the individual cells was much greater. It was increased in both cytoplasm and nucleus and there was a great increase of the reaction in the cell membranes. These reactions were also increased in the other cells of the cortex (fig. 10).

Submaxillary Gland

Ethanolamine-phosphate at pH 9.0 was the substrate used here. In the young animal the reaction was intense in the nuclei of the

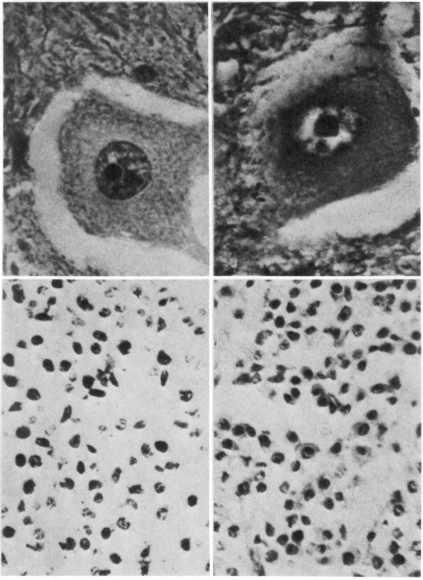

Fig. 5 Fig. 6

Fig. 7 Fig. 8

Fig. 5. Cell from region of origin of motor root of 5th nerve, in young animal. *Substrate:* ethanolamine-phosphate.

Fig. 6. Cell from region of origin of motor root of 5th nerve, in old animal. *Substrate:* ethanolamine-phosphate.

Fig. 7. Anterior pituitary. Young animal. *Substrate:* oestrone-phosphate.

Fig. 8. Anterior pituitary. Old animal. *Substrate:* oestrone-phosphate.

116

Fig. 9   Fig. 10

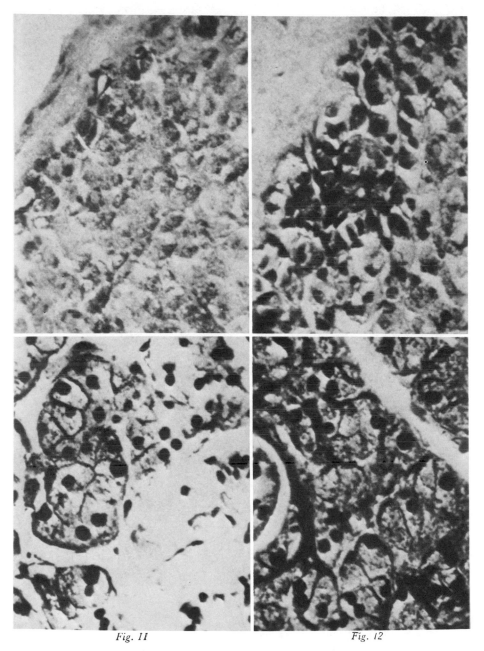

Fig. 11   Fig. 12

Fig. 9. Adrenal cortex. Young animal. *Substrate:* pyridoxal-phosphate (pH 9.0)
Fig. 10. Adrenal cortex. Old animal. *Substrate:* pyridoxal-phosphate (pH 9.0).
Fig. 11. Sub-maxillary gland. Young animal. *Substrate:* ethanolamine-phosphate.
Fig. 12. Sub-maxillary gland. Old animal. *Substrate:* ethanolamine-phosphate.

Fig. 13 Fig. 14

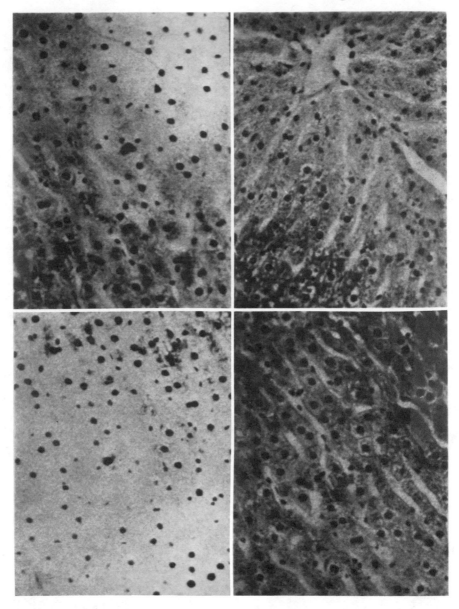

Fig. 15   Fig. 16

Fig. 13. Liver young animal. *Substrate:* carbamyl-phosphate.
Fig. 14. Liver old animal. *Substrate:* carbamyl-phosphate.
Fig. 15. Liver young animal. *Substrate:* oestrone-phosphate.
Fig. 16. Liver old animal. *Substrate:* oestrone-phosphate.

acinar cells and in their cell membranes. A slight granular reaction was present in the cytoplasm (fig. 11).

In the old animals these cytoplasmic and membrane reactions were greatly increased but the nuclear reaction did not appear to change (fig. 12).

Liver

Carbamyl-phosphate and oestrone-phosphate at pH 9.0 gave the following results. With both substrates the reaction in young animals was largely nuclear although many cells showed a cytoplasmic reaction with carbamyl-phosphate (figs. 14 and 15).

In the old animals there was a general increase in cytoplasmic reaction with carbamyl-phosphate it was obviously located in small well-defined cytoplasmic bodies (fig. 13). With oestrone-phosphate this increased reaction appeared to be mostly diffused through the cytoplasm (fig. 16).

Discussion

So far as is known at present oestrone- and cortisone-phosphates are not formed in the chemical processes involved in the *in vivo* metabolism of these compounds although it may well be shown in the future that they are. It may be however that increased hydrolysis of these compounds is an aspect of the increased dephosphorylating activity of old tissues. On the other hand of the remaining three, two (pyridoxal-phosphate and carbamyl-phosphate) are metabolically important substances while the role of the third (ethanolamine-phosphate), although it is widely distributed in the body, has not yet been elucidated; it may be associated with phospholipid metabolism. Pyridoxyl-phosphate forms the prosthetic group of several and possibly all amino-acid decarboxylases; carbamyl-phosphate is an important intermediary in urea synthesis in the body, it acts as a carbamyl donor in a variety of enzymatic systems. The fact that these substances are more easily dephosphorylated in old tissues may be of considerable significance since it may indicate a shift in the balance between synthesis and hydrolysis of these physiologically very important substances towards the latter.

It is of interest that *Byrbye* and *Kirk* (1956) and *Zorzoli* (1955) have shown an increase of β-glucuronidase and acid phosphatase in the cells of older animal.

De Duve et al. (1955) have described a series of bodies in rat liver cells which appear to be microsomes and in which most of the hydrolytic emzymes appear to be concentrated. Among these enzymes were β-glucuronidase, acid phosphatase, cathepsin and ribonuclease; the bodies were named "lysosomes". De Duve claimed that the unrestricted activity of these bodies after death was due to tissue autolysis. An increase in activity of these bodies in old tissues either by loss of inhibitory control or otherwise may help to explain the progressive inefficiency and degeneration of tissues as they age. It may for example be the explanation of the degeneration and loss of neurones from the brain in older animals.

Summary

There is a general increase of dephosphorylating activity in the cells of old animals particularly in the cytoplasm.

References

Byrbye, M., and J. E. Kirk: J. Geront. 11, 33, 1956.
De Duve, C., et al.: Biochem. J. 60, 604, 1955.
Zorzoli, A.: J. Geront. 10, 156, 1955.

Oxidative Phosphorylation in Mitochondria from Aged Rats*

Eugene C. Weinbach and Joel Garbus

With the Technical Assistance of C. Elwood Claggett

Studies of oxidative phosphorylation as related to the age of the organism serve a twofold purpose. On the one hand, they may contribute to our understanding of the mechanisms of oxidative phosphorylation by introducing aging *in vivo* as an experimental variable, and on the other hand, such studies add to our knowledge of the biochemical changes associated with physiological aging. In a previous report we have shown that the levels of oxidation of β-hydroxybutyrate and the concomitant phosphorylation are significantly lower in liver mitochondria of aged rats (1). The present paper amplifies the earlier observations, and in addition summarizes studies of such ancillary factors as mitochondrial stability, the P_i-ATP[1] exchange reaction, and nucleotide content of liver and brain.

EXPERIMENTAL

Animals—Sprague-Dawley rats from a colony especially maintained to study aging were employed. Purina laboratory chow, supplemented weekly with fresh fruits and vegetables, horse meat, and milk, was fed *ad libitum*. Animals 24-months-old or more were considered aged in this study. Every experiment included as a control a 3- to 4-month-old rat treated identical to that described for the aged animal.

The animals were killed by decapitation, and the brain and liver were immediately and simultaneously excised and placed in chilled 0.25 M sucrose (4°). Only tissues which appeared grossly free from disease were used.

* Presented in part before the Fourth International Congress of Gerontology at Merano, Italy, July 14 to 19, 1957.

[1] The abbreviation used is: P_i, inorganic orthophosphate.

Mitochondria—Liver mitochondria were isolated by differential centrifugation in 0.25 M sucrose essentially by the procedure of Schneider (2), with the precautions to be described in detail elsewhere. Mitochondria prepared in this manner displayed a high degree of stability with respect to oxidative phosphorylation (3). Isolation of brain mitochondria was accomplished by adapting a procedure described for mouse brain (4). The brain was quickly removed, its volume recorded, and a 10 per cent homogenate prepared in 0.25 M sucrose. Unbroken cells, nuclei, debris, and some mitochondria were removed by centrifuging the homogenate at 8000 $\times$ g at 0° for 2 minutes, including the time necessary to bring the rotor to full speed. The supernatant fluid was transferred by chilled pipette to prechilled tubes and centrifuged at 20,000 $\times$ g for 20 minutes. The pellet thus obtained was washed by resuspension in a volume of cold 0.25 M sucrose equal to twice the original volume of the brain. After recentrifugation at 20,000 $\times$ g for 20 minutes, the pellet was suspended as before. Each milliliter of the final suspensions represented the mitochondria of 0.5 gm., wet weight, of liver or brain tissue.

The concentrations of all mitochondrial suspensions were determined before use by measurements of their turbidities at 520 mμ in the Beckman model DU spectrophotometer and by estimation of their protein content by the biuret reaction. On the basis of these measurements the suspensions were adjusted to assure the use of essentially equal amounts of mitochondria from old and young tissue in each comparative experiment. However, it should be emphasized that all data are calculated on the basis of the final content of mitochondrial nitrogen (micro-Kjeldahl).

Analytical—Oxidative phosphorylation (1) and ATPase activity (5) were determined as previously described. Total nucleotides were extracted from mitochondria with cold 1.5 N perchloric acid according to Siekevitz and Potter (6) and the absorption determined at 260 mμ. Pyridine nucleotides were determined by the single extraction procedure of Spirtes and Eichel (7). The extracts of whole liver tissue were centrifuged at 100,000 $\times$ g for 1 hour before optical measurements were made. This was necessitated by the high turbidity present in the extracts of livers of the aged rats. In a few experiments fluorometric measurements of the pyridine nucleotide content of mitochondria also were made (8). The observation that extracts of whole liver tissue of the aged rat contained substances which were inherently highly fluorescent precluded accurate fluorometric assay with whole tissues.

The technique for determining the P_i-ATP exchange reaction was based on the method of Cooper and Lehninger (9). P_i and ATP were separated (10) and aliquots counted in a Tracerlab automatic gas flow counter.

Routinely all determinations were performed in duplicate or triplicate.

RESULTS

Gross Properties of Tissues and Mitochondria—The tissues and mitochondria from the old animals differed both in color and consistency from those of the young. The liver from the aged rat was paler, more fibrous, and of a firmer texture than that from the young. These differences especially were evident when the tissues were pulped. Mitochondria isolated from liver of the older animals were more heavily pigmented and showed a marked tendency to adhere to the centrifuge tube as a viscous pellet. The supernatant fraction remaining after isolation of the mitochondria also was more heavily colored. Absorption spectra of the supernatant fractions revealed that this difference between young and old animals was of a quantitative rather than a qualitative nature.[2] Another gross difference in these preparations was that the fatty layer which moved centripetally during the isolation of liver mitochondria always was more abundant with the older tissue. Whole brain tissue and mitochondria displayed similar age-related differences in color and consistency, although not to the same extent.

Oxidative Phosphorylation—The data summarized in Table I show that brain mitochondria from the aged animals exhibited no decline in their capacity for oxidative phosphorylation with succinate as substrate. Although other substrates were not extensively explored,[3] a few experiments with α-ketoglutarate and glutamate also indicated no age-related differences. These findings are analogous to our earlier work with fortified brain homogenates (1) in which there was no decline in oxidative phosphorylation with age.[4]

---

[2] The supernatant fractions remaining after mitochondrial sedimentation were centrifuged at 20,000 $\times$ g for 30 minutes. These "cleared" fractions were diluted 10-fold with H_2O and their absorption spectra determined. Both preparations absorbed maximally at 415 mμ.

[3] β-Hydroxybutyrate was not used as a substrate for oxidative phosphorylation with brain mitochondria, because it is poorly oxidized and acetoacetic acid, the oxidation product, does not accumulate stoichiometrically in brain tissue.

[4] These findings are of interest in light of recent studies *in vivo* of normal old men, in whom cerebral blood flow and oxygen consumption were measured. No age-related changes were found (11).

TABLE I

TABLE I

Effect of age on oxidative phosphorylation with brain mitochondria

The figures are averages of 10 experiments. Each flask contained, in a final volume of 3 ml., 30 μmoles of tris(hydroxymethyl)aminomethane buffer, pH 7.4; 20 μmoles of orthophosphate, pH 7.4; 30 μmoles of succinate; 20 μmoles of $MgCl_2$; 4 μmoles of ATP; 0.5 μmole of DPN; 0.035 μmole of cytochrome c; 150 μmoles of glucose; 0.5 mg. of hexokinase (Sigma Chemical Company, Type II); 40 μmoles of KF (added last); and 0.5 ml. (0.95 mg. N, average) of mitochondria. Incubated in air for 30 minutes at 30°.

Age	ΔP_i	ΔO	P:O
	$\mu moles/mg.$ N	$\mu\ atoms/mg.$ N	
Young (3 to 4 months).........	14.6	8.5	1.7
Old (24 months or older).......	14.2	8.2	1.7

On the other hand, significant declines were found in the levels of both substrate oxidation (-39 per cent) and concomitant phosphorylation (-37 per cent), when β-hydroxybutyrate was oxidized by liver mitochondria from aged animals (Table II). Little or no age-related differences in either activity were observed when succinate, α-ketoglutarate, glutamate, or malate were used as substrates. However, stability studies, to be described below, revealed that age-related differences in the utilization of these substrates do develop after prolonged storage of the mitochondria.

Stability Studies—Earlier we had suggested that the declines in oxidative phosphorylation noted in liver mitochondria from the aged rat may in part be attributed to an increased fragility of these preparations (1). This now has been tested by subjecting the isolated liver mitochondria to various deleterious procedures such as freezing and thawing, preincubation at 37° in the absence of added substrate, and the presence of high concentrations of pentachlorophenol (5). Mitochondrial swelling as measured by changes in optical density was used as a gross index of physical stability. Evaluations of oxidative phosphorylation and of ATPase activity were made to detect changes in enzymatic stability. Such studies revealed that the mitochondria from aged rats were somewhat more sensitive to these deleterious treatments than those of the younger animals (Fig. 1; Table III).

Stability of Oxidative Phosphorylation—Experiments with young animals have shown that liver mitochondria, when isolated under carefully controlled conditions, retain their capacity for oxidative phosphorylation after prolonged storage at 4° (3). It was of interest to determine whether mitochondria

Table II

Effect of age on oxidative phosphorylation with liver mitochondria

Each flask contained, in a final volume of 2 ml., 80 μmoles of glycylglycine buffer, pH 7.4; 50 μmoles of DL-β-hydroxybutyrate or 20 μmoles of other substrates; 20 or 30 μmoles of orthophosphate, pH 7.4; 5 μmoles of ADP; 2 μmoles of DPN; 0.03 μmole of cytochrome c; 50 μmoles of glucose; 0.5 mg. of hexokinase (Sigma Chemical Company, Type II); 10 μmoles of $MgCl_2$; 30 μmoles of KF (added last), and 0.5 ml. (0.9 mg. N, average) of mitochondria. Experiments with α-ketoglutarate and glutamate included 20 μmoles of malonate. Oxidation of β-hydroxybutyrate was followed by measuring the stoichiometric accumulation of aceto-acetate (12). Incubated in air for 20 minutes at 30°.

Age*	No. of experiments	Substrate	ΔP_i	ΔO	P:O
			$\mu moles/$ mg. N	μ atoms/ mg. N	
Young	8	β-Hydroxybutyrate	17.2	5.9	2.9
Old		β-Hydroxybutyrate	10.8	3.6	3.0
Young	3	β-Hydroxybutyrate†	16.4	5.5	3.0
Old		β-Hydroxybutyrate†	11.4	3.4	3.3
Young	3	Succinate	21.1	11.1	1.9
Old		Succinate	21.6	10.9	2.0
Young	3	α-Ketoglutarate	21.4	5.7	3.8
Old		α-Ketoglutarate	21.4	5.6	3.8
Young	2	Glutamate	19.0	7.8	2.4
Old		Glutamate	19.0	7.2	2.6
Young	2	Malate	17.4	8.4	2.0
Old		Malate	14.9	8.3	1.8

* Young, 3 to 4 months; old, 24 months or older.

† Each flask also contained 6 mg. of crystallized bovine plasma albumin (Armour).

from the aged rats displayed this same stability. The data assembled in Table IV, indeed, show that although the mitochondria from the aged rat retain their capacity for oxidative phosphorylation under these conditions, differences in their stability become evident. Even though little change occurred after the first 24 hours of storage, a differential decline in both phosphorylation and the P:O ratios was observed after 48 hours,

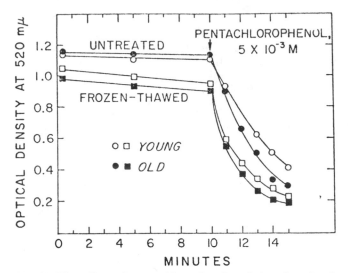

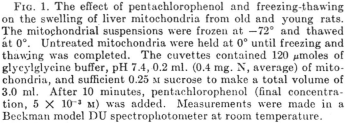

FIG. 1. The effect of pentachlorophenol and freezing-thawing on the swelling of liver mitochondria from old and young rats. The mitochondrial suspensions were frozen at −72° and thawed at 0°. Untreated mitochondria were held at 0° until freezing and thawing was completed. The cuvettes contained 120 μmoles of glycylglycine buffer, pH 7.4, 0.2 ml. (0.4 mg. N, average) of mitochondria, and sufficient 0.25 M sucrose to make a total volume of 3.0 ml. After 10 minutes, pentachlorophenol (final concentration, 5 × 10⁻³ M) was added. Measurements were made in a Beckman model DU spectrophotometer at room temperature.

and progressed to marked differences between the preparations from the old and young rats after 72 hours. These differences were most evident in preparations which had been sampled daily. Mitochondria left undisturbed until final assay still exhibited age-related declines in both oxidation and phosphorylation but displayed little age-related differences in the P:O ratios. Thus, the most striking age-related differences were found with mitochondrial suspensions with activity impaired by prolonged storage plus the mechanical attrition induced by repeated sampling. For example, after 72 hours of storage the phosphate uptake of the samples which had been assayed repeatedly declined 84 per cent with mitochondria from the aged rat, but the corresponding decline in the young rat preparations was only 38 per cent. It may be recalled that freshly isolated liver mitochondria from the aged rat showed no decline in the levels of oxidative phosphorylation when succinate was used as substrate (Table II). However, after 48 hours of storage the mitochondria from the aged rat were impaired in their use of this substrate to a greater extent than were the preparations from the younger rats (Table IV). This may reflect a metabolic

TABLE III
Oxidative phosphorylation with frozen-thawed or preincubated liver mitochondria

The reaction medium was the same as given in Table II. Freezing and thawing were accomplished as described in Fig. 1. Preincubation at 37° for 30 minutes. The untreated mitochondria were held at 0° during these procedures.

Age*	Substrate	Treatment	ΔP_i ($\mu moles/mg. N$)	ΔO ($\mu atoms/mg. N$)	P:O
Experiment A					
Young.....	β-Hydroxybutyrate	Untreated	17.2	5.9	2.9
Old	β-Hydroxybutyrate	Untreated	10.8	3.6	3.0
Young.....	β-Hydroxybutyrate	Frozen-thawed	12.5	7.8	1.6
Old........	β-Hydroxybutyrate	Frozen-thawed	4.9	3.7	1.3
Young.....	β-Hydroxybutyrate	Preincubated	13.7	6.3	2.2
Old........	β-Hydroxybutyrate	Preincubated	7.7	3.3	2.3
Experiment B					
Young.....	Succinate	Untreated	21.1	11.1	1.9
Old........	Succinate	Untreated	21.6	10.9	2.0
Young.....	Succinate	Preincubated	15.9	15.6	1.0
Old........	Succinate	Preincubated	15.3	15.2	1.0
Experiment C					
Young.....	β-Hydroxybutyrate	DPN omitted	17.4	5.3	3.2
Old........	β-Hydroxybutyrate	DPN omitted	12.0	3.8	3.2
Young.....	β-Hydroxybutyrate	Preincubated, DPN omitted	12.0	4.5	2.7
Old........	β-Hydroxybutyrate	Preincubated, DPN omitted	7.7	3.0	2.6

* Young, 3 to 4 months; old, 24 months or older.

TABLE IV

Effect of storage of liver mitochondria on oxidative phosphorylation

Experimental conditions as in Table II. Suspensions of mitochondria were stored at 4° until assayed at the times shown. Samples were either assayed daily or left undisturbed as indicated.

Age*	No. of experiments	Substrate	Time of storage	Previously sampled	ΔP_i	ΔO	P:O
			hrs.		$\mu moles/ mg. N$	$\mu atoms/ mg. N$	
Young	8	β-Hydroxybutyrate	0		17.2	5.9	2.9
Old					10.8	3.6	3.0
Young	4	β-Hydroxybutyrate	24	Yes	19.0	7.1	2.7
Old					10.5	4.0	2.6
Young	3	β-Hydroxybutyrate	48	Yes	14.5	7.2	2.0
Old					4.4	3.5	1.3
Young	3	β-Hydroxybutyrate	48	No	16.2	5.5	2.9
Old					8.8	3.0	2.9
Young	3	β-Hydroxybutyrate	72	Yes	10.7	6.4	1.6
Old					1.7	2.7	0.6
Young	3	β-Hydroxybutyrate	72	No	13.6	7.5	1.2
Old					5.2	3.6	1.4
Young	3	Succinate	24	Yes	18.0	10.2	1.8
Old					18.5	10.2	1.8
Young	3	Succinate	48	Yes	18.0	12.9	1.4
Old					15.3	14.2	1.1
Young	2	α-Ketoglutarate	24	No	13.5	3.5	3.9
Old					15.1	3.9	3.9
Young	2	Malate	48	No	12.5	6.6	1.9
Old					10.0	5.8	1.7

* Young, 3 to 4 months; old, 24 months or older.

inadequacy inherent in the mitochondrial enzymatic organization of the aged animal. Such a defect may not be apparent in fresh preparations which display high phosphorylative activity when assayed under conditions designed for maximal phosphorylation.

Bovine albumin, which has been shown to increase mitochondrial stability (13, 14) did not restore the metabolic activity of liver mitochondria of the aged rats to the level found with the younger animals (Table II).

The possibility that liver mitochondria from aged animals contain a substance inhibitory to the oxidation of β-hydroxybutyrate was tested by combining mitochondria from both age groups and determining the levels of oxidative phosphorylation in the mixture. A depression in these levels would be anticipated if the old tissue contained a diffusible endogenous inhibitor. In the experiments with combined mitochondria no decline was observed, a finding which suggests that the presence of such an inhibitor is unlikely.

ATPase Activity—The experiments summarized in the data of Table V revealed no age-related differences in the ATPase

TABLE V

Adenosinetriphosphatase activity in liver and brain mitochondria

The assay medium contained 40 μmoles of glycylglycine buffer, pH 7.4; 5 μmoles of $MgCl_2$; 6 μmoles of ATP; 0.2 ml. (0.4 mg. of N, average) of mitochondria plus pentachlorophenol as indicated; and sufficient 0.25 M sucrose to make a final volume of 1.0 ml. Incubated for 10 minutes at 25°.

Mitochondria	Treatment	ΔP_i	
		Young*	Old*
		μmoles/ mg. N	
Brain	Untreated (control)	6.7	6.7
	Pentachlorophenol, 5×10^{-5} M	7.0	7.2
	Pentachlorophenol, 5×10^{-4} M	4.6	4.8
Liver	Untreated (control)	0.30	0.34
	Pentachlorophenol, 5×10^{-5} M	8.0	6.6
	Preincubated†	3.1	3.5
	Preincubated + pentachlorophenol, 5×10^{-4} M	1.2	1.8
	Frozen and thawed	4.8	5.2
	Frozen and thawed + pentachlorophenol, 5×10^{-5} M	8.0	7.9

* Young, 3 to 4 months; old, 24 months or older.
† Preincubation at 37° for 30 minutes.

activity of freshly isolated brain or liver mitochondria. Likewise, the response of mitochondria of the aged rat to various experimental procedures known to influence this activity did not materially differ from that exhibited by the corresponding mitochondrial preparations of younger animals.

P_i-ATP Exchange Reaction—Rat liver mitochondria catalyze a rapid exchange between P_i and ATP (15). In Table VI it can be seen that the mitochondria from the aged animals were equally as effective in catalyzing this reaction as those from the younger animals. Brain mitochondria, on the other hand, were not very active in promoting the exchange reaction, possibly because of their high ATPase activity (Table V). However, similarly to liver mitochondria, they displayed no marked differences associated with age. As in the case of oxidative phosphorylation, age-related differences became evident after storage of the liver mitochondria at low temperatures (Table VI).

Nucleotide Levels—Because of the lessened ability of liver mitochondria of the aged rat to metabolize β-hydroxybutyrate, a substrate the oxidation of which is mediated through pyridine nucleotide, and since nucleotides in general have an important

TABLE VI

P_i-ATP exchange reaction with liver and brain mitochondria

The reaction medium contained, in 1 ml., 10 μmoles of tris(hydroxymethyl)aminomethane buffer, pH 7.4; 6 μmoles of ATP, 6 μmoles of potassium phosphate labeled with P^{32} (initially, 100,000 c.p.m.); and 0.2 ml. (0.4 mg. N, average) of mitochondria. Final pH, 6.9. The reaction was terminated after 10 minutes by the addition of 0.1 ml. of 25 per cent perchloric acid. Temperature, 30°.

Age*	No. of experiments	Experimental Conditions	P_i exchanged
			μmoles/mg. N
Young.......	9	Liver mitochondria,	4.8
Old..........		freshly isolated	4.8
Young.......	2	Liver mitochondria,	4.5
Old..........		24 hrs. storage at 4°	3.7
Young.......	2	Liver mitochondria,	0.7
Old..........		48 hrs. storage at 4°	None
Young.......	7	Brain mitochondria,	0.88
Old..........		freshly isolated	0.83

* Young, 3 to 4 months; old, 24 months or older.

function in oxidative phosphorylation, it was of interest to estimate their levels in the tissues of the aged animals. As shown in Table VII, the total acid-soluble nucleotide content of mitochondria from both liver and brain, determined by the absorption at 260 mμ, was significantly lower in the aged animal. Siekevitz and Potter (6) have shown that the acid-soluble material absorbing maximally at 260 mμ consists mainly of adenine nucleotides. However, the levels of pyridine nucleotides, also present in these acid extracts, were lower in the brain and liver of the old rat as determined by enzymatic assay. The content of oxidized DPN was found to be less in both whole tissue and mitochondria of these organs (Table VII). The possibility that there are fewer cells in the liver and brain of the aged rat could account for the lower level of DPN found in the whole tissue. Such an explanation, however, appears unlikely since the DPN content of mitochondria when expressed on a nitrogen basis also was lower. Although the relationship between age and the content of DPNH is somewhat less certain, owing to difficulties in measurement of the latter (*cf.* (16)), the data suggest that DPNH levels also may be altered in the aged rat. In liver mitochondria and whole brain tissue of the aged rat these levels were lower. The high content of DPNH found in whole liver tissue of the aged animal is puzzling and may reflect either the presence of substances reacting non-specifically in the enzymatic assay ((17), page 98) or a shift in the ratio of oxidized

TABLE VII

Age and nucleotide content of mitochondria and whole tissue

The figures in parentheses refer to the number of experiments. DPN and DPNH were determined enzymatically and total DPN + TPN, fluorometrically. See the text. DPN of 92 per cent purity and DPNH of 88 per cent purity (Sigma) were used as standards.

Tissue Preparation	Age*	E_{260} per mg. N	DPN	DPNH	DPN + TPN
			$\mu mg./mg.\ N$		
Liver mitochondria	Young	0.713(8)	9.7(4)	29.5(4)	16.6(3)
	Old	0.632(8)	7.9(4)	24.2(4)	9.6(3)
Brain mitochondria	Young	0.498(5)	11.8(3)	None (3)	9.9(3)
	Old	0.435(5)	9.9(3)	None (3)	8.7(3)
Whole liver†	Young		376(7)	384(7)	
	Old		251(7)	507(7)	
Whole brain†	Young		133(6)	67(6)	
	Old		110(6)	47(6)	

* Young, 3 to 4 months; old, 24 months or older.
† Values are in μgm. per gm. of tissue.

131

to reduced nucleotides in the whole liver tissue of the aged rat. Possible inaccuracies in estimating the absolute values of pyridine nucleotides introduced by a single extraction procedure have been suggested (16, 18). However, this in no way invalidates the age-related differences observed, since such differences, rather than the evaluation of absolute levels of pyridine nucleotides, were the objective in these experiments.

In view of the lowered levels of nucleotides observed in mitochondria from the aged rat, DPN was omitted from the reaction medium used for oxidative phosphorylation. This was done to evaluate the rather remote possibility that the deficiency in the oxidation of β-hydroxybutyrate might be exaggerated by the omission of this nucleotide. As shown in Table III, Experiment C, the omission of DPN did not alter the utilization of β-hydroxybutyrate either in fresh or preincubated mitochondria from animals of both age groups. These findings are concordant with the generally accepted view that only the mitochondrially-bound DPN is functional in electron transport.

Liver mitochondrial suspensions were incubated at 37°, and the release of acid-soluble material absorbing maximally at 260 mμ was studied as an additional index of possible age differences. The data in Table VIII show the partition of this material between the mitochondrial pellets and supernatant fractions before and after incubation. As in the case of the total acid-soluble nucleotide content of the mitochondria (Table VII), the mitochondria from the aged rat yielded significantly lower total values. This decrement was accounted for entirely by the lesser

TABLE VIII

Nucleotide release upon incubation of liver mitochondria

The figures are average values of three experiments expressed as optical densities at 260 mμ corrected for mitochondrial nitrogen. Technique as described in reference (6).

	Pellet	Supernatant fraction	Total
Freshly isolated			
Young	0.677	0.062	0.739
Old........................	0.577	0.062	0.639
After incubation†			
Young.....................	0.392	0.338	0.730
Old........................	0.329	0.323	0.652

* Young, 3 to 4 months; old, 24 months or older.

† Incubated at 37° for 30 minutes in absence of exogenous substrate.

132

amount of material absorbing at 260 mμ found in the pellet (Table VIII). During incubation, the amount of nucleotide release in both suspensions was the same (approximately 43 per cent), indicating that liver mitochondria of the aged rat were not uniquely susceptible to nucleotide loss under these conditions.

DISCUSSION

Although the decline in metabolic activity associated with age has been amply documented for many organisms (19), the physiological basis for this decline remains a matter of conjecture. This decreased activity has been ascribed to a loss of cells, a decline in the metabolism of individual cells, or a combination of these factors (20). Since isolated mitochondria represent an organized complement of enzymes of which activity can be assayed independently of the cellular environment or cell number, they provide a convenient tool for investigating possible changes in metabolic activities with age. Indeed, studies reported here with liver mitochondria from the aged rat revealed a decrement in their capacity for oxidative phosphorylation when β-hydroxybutyrate was used as substrate (Table II). Green and coworkers (21), in studies with fragmented mitochondria, have shown that β-hydroxybutyric acid dehydrogenase and certain other pyridinoprotein enzymes are intimately associated in a submitochondrial entity which the investigators have designated the "phosphorylating electron transport particle." Our studies with freshly isolated, intact mitochondria revealed that oxidative phosphorylation did not decline with age when α-ketoglutarate, glutamate, and malate were used as substrates, in contrast to the decline observed with β-hydroxybutyrate (Table II). If the decreased β-hydroxybutyrate utilization is related to the lowered levels of pyridine nucleotides found in the liver mitochondria of the aged rat (Table VII), it is puzzling that a similar decrement was not found with other substrates oxidized by pyridinoprotein enzymes in the mitochondrial entity associated with β-hydroxybutyric acid dehydrogenase. These observations may imply that the passage of electrons and concomitant phosphorylations with β-hydroxybutyrate is via an age-sensitive pathway which differs from that utilized by the other substrates. Thus the use of mitochondria from aged animals reveals facets of oxidative phosphorylation not evident in preparations from the younger animals which are conventionally employed.

The data of Table VI, showing no age-related differences in the activities of the enzymes which catalyze the P_i-ATP exchange, indicate that enzymes other than those involved in a terminal transphosphorylation sequence are probable sites of the observed deficiences in oxidative phosphorylation.

Consideration of all data reported here relating to mitochondrial stability (Tables III to VI and VIII and Fig. 1) indicates that liver mitochondria isolated from the aged rat are, indeed, more sensitive to injurious experimental procedures than those from the young. However, it should be noted that age-related differences in stability become pronounced and patently obvious only with increasing severity of these procedures (Table IV). The age-related differences in mitochondrial stability observed with carefully isolated fresh liver mitochondria are minimal and cannot account for the lowered levels of oxidative phosphorylation. This view is supported by the following considerations. (a) Increased fragility of mitochondria is associated with uncoupling of phosphorylation from oxidation rather than equivalent decreases in both activities. (b) It would be anticipated that all dehydrogenases involved in oxidative phosphorylation would be equally affected. This was not the case (Table II). (c) Studies of physical stability of carefully isolated fresh mitochondria show little difference in the initial fragility of mitochondria from both age groups. An alternative and more likely possibility is that the differences in mitochondrial metabolism described in this report are true reflections of altered enzymatic activities associated with physiological aging.

SUMMARY

1. Brain and liver tissue and mitochondria from the aged rat displayed gross physical differences, such as in color and consistency, when compared with the tissues of the young animal.

2. Oxidative phosphorylation with β-hydroxybutyrate as the substrate declined in liver mitochondria from aged rats. Although similar decrements were not seen with other substrates such as succinate and α-ketoglutarate in fresh preparations, age-related differences were evident after prolonged storage of the mitochondria at 4° and other pretreatments. As found previously with homogenates, brain mitochondria did not show any age-associated declines in oxidative phosphorylation with succinate as substrate.

3. Stability studies revealed that liver mitochondria isolated from older animals are more sensitive to deleterious experimental procedures, as evaluated by physical and enzymatic techniques. This sensitivity increased with the severity of the treatment. However, mitochondrial fragility alone does not account for the age-associated declines in oxidative phosphorylation observed with fresh preparations.

4. Measurements of the inorganic orthophosphate-adenosine triphosphate exchange revealed no differences in activity between age groups, thus precluding a transphosphorylation sequence as the site of the observed decline in oxidative phosphorylation.

5. Lowered contents of pyridine and adenine nucleotides were found in the mitochondria of the aged rat. This may be related to the impaired oxidative phosphorylation.

6. Consideration of these observations suggest that there is a true age-related deficit in oxidative phosphorylation with certain substrates and that this deficit occurs early in the sequence of electron transport.

REFERENCES

1. WEINBACH, E. C., AND GARBUS, J., Nature, 178, 1225 (1956).
2. SCHNEIDER, W. C., in W. W. UMBREIT, R. H. BURRIS, AND J. F. STAUFFER, Manometric techniques and tissue metabolism, Burgess Publishing Company, Minneapolis, 1949, p. 148.
3. WEINBACH, E. C., Federation Proc., 16, 268 (1957).
4. DUBUY, H. G., AND HESSELBACH, M. L., J. Histochem. Cytochem., 4, 363 (1956)
5. WEINBACH, E. C., J. Biol. Chem., 221, 609 (1956).
6. SIEKEVITZ, P., AND POTTER, V. R., J. Biol. Chem., 215, 221 (1955).
7. ORTES, M. A., AND EICHEL, H. J., Arch. Biochem. Biophys., 53, 308 (1954).
8. CIOTTI, M. M., AND KAPLAN, N. O., in S. P. COLOWICK AND N. O. KAPLAN (Editors), Methods in enzymology, Vol. III, Academic Press, Inc., New York, 1957, p. 890.
9. COOPER, C., AND LEHNINGER, A. L., J. Biol. Chem., 224, 561 (1957).
10. NIELSEN, S. O., AND LEHNINGER, A. L., J. Biol. Chem., 215, 555 (1955).
11. SOKOLOFF, L., in J. E. BIRREN, H. IMUS, AND W. WINDLE, The process of aging in the nervous system, Charles C Thomas, Springfield, Illinois, in press.
12. WALKER, P. G., Biochem. J., 58, 699 (1954).
13. SACKTOR, B., J. Gen. Physiol., 37, 343 (1954).
14. PULLMAN, M. G., AND RACKER, E., Science, 123, 1105 (1956).
15. BOYER, P. D., FALCONE, A. B., AND HARRISON, W. H., Nature, 174, 401 (1954).
16. JEDEIKIN, L. A., AND WEINHOUSE, S., J. Biol. Chem., 213, 271 (1955).
17. SINGER, T. P., AND KEARNEY, E. B., Advances in Enzymol., 15, 79 (1954).
18. GLOCK, G. E., AND McLEAN, P., Biochem. J., 61, 388 (1955).
19. COMFORT, A., The biology of senescence, Rinehart and Company, Inc., New York, 1956.
20. BARROWS, C. H., JR., Federation Proc., 15, 954 (1956).
21. GREEN, D. E., The Harvey lectures, Series 52, (1956–1957), Academic Press, Inc., New York, 1958, p. 177.

Vasculature

STUDIES ON THE AGE-RELATED CHANGES OCCURRING IN HUMAN CEREBRAL ARTERIES

C. VELICAN

SUMMARY

From the 4th to the 7th decades of life, the period in which cerebral atherosclerosis increases in frequency and severity, the macromolecules and macromolecular complexes of the intimal connective tissue of the lesion-free specimens of cerebral arteries undergo spontaneous modifications, reflected by changes in: chemical components, reactive groups, electrical charge, susceptibility to enzymatic digestions and chemical extractions. These age-related changes determine: (i) the differentiation in the newly formed intimal connective tissue of two sublayers, displaying a distinct pattern of macromolecular composition, organization and aggregation; (ii) the increase, in the outer intimal sublayer, of various cross-links between carbohydrates, non-collagen proteins, elastin and collagen macromolecules, resulting in an abnormal state of aggregation which prevents enzyme–substrate interactions, *in vitro*, on tissue sections; (iii) the transformation of some limited areas of the inner intimal sublayer into a loose-mucoid and edematous tissue process which seems to be preceded by a spontaneous and progressive dissolution of some constituents of the ground substance, reticular, elastic and collagen fibers; (iv) the diminution of the histochemical reactivity of the sulfate groups, due to a progressive blockade of these radicals by basic proteins.

Key words: *Aging – Atherosclerosis – Cerebral arteries – Macromolecular composition, organization and aggregation*

INTRODUCTION

"The most dramatic aspect of cerebrovascular disease is its relationship to age, which is one of a logarithmic increase"[1]. This assertion is supported by numerous clinical, pathological and biochemical data[2-9]. In all studies on this subject, both hemorrhage and thrombosis become strikingly more common the older the group investigated. Major differences in prognosis for thrombosis are also strongly age related. In the light of these findings, some authors believe that cerebral atherosclerosis appears to be preventable only to the extent that we could reverse the aging process[1].

Morphological attempts to analyze the age-related changes of the human cerebral arteries which could favor the development of atherosclerosis are very few. The first reports on this topic have revealed a loss of elastic fibers and a gradual increase in collagen fibers at the expense of the medial muscle cells with increasing age[10-12]. Other papers stressed the alterations of the internal elastic membrane, as well as the accumulation of metachromatic material at the sites of reduplication and fragmentation[13-15].

The unique histochemical analysis on the age-related changes in the cerebral arteries, found as published data in the available literature[16-18], pointed out the existence of a slightly different pattern of acid mucopolysaccharides in fetuses, infants, young juveniles and adults. It is reflected, for instance, by the presence in fetuses, infants and young juveniles of acid mucopolysaccharides hydrolyzable with testicular hyaluronidase; whereas in the adults a resistance to the same enzyme was noted. The ratio of chrondroitin-sulfate B to chondroitin-sulfate A and/or C increased with age and with severe changes in the internal elastic membrane. Concomitantly there was an increase in the ratio of coarse collagen to fine collagen. The close association of chondroitin-sulfate B with coarse collagen and/or fragmentation and/or reduplication of the internal elastic membrane was considered as a reinforcement mechanism to strengthen the arterial wall.

The present paper is an attempt to give a further insight into the age-related changes occurring in the cerebral arteries and to correlate these age-related changes with the progressive development of cerebral atherosclerosis.

MATERIALS AND METHODS

The results of the present studies are based on the histochemical analysis of 300 samples of human intracranial arteries. After being dissected from the base of the brain, the circle of Willis with 2 cm of attached anterior, posterior and middle cerebral basilar artery and 1 cm of each vertebral artery was laid out on a wet paper towel[19]. Samples of 0.5 cm have been taken from each cerebral artery, sectioned perpendicularly to the longitudinal axis of the vessel.

In order to avoid or to minimize the oxidizing effect of various fixatives and their influence on constitutive substances, reactive groups and cross-linkage of macromolecules, we have used in this work: (i) unfixed specimens, cut at —20°C in a cryostat and (ii) specimens fixed in Carnoy's fluid (absolute ethyl alcohol–chloroform–glacial acetic acid, 60 : 30 : 10, v/v/v). The solution was prepared at the time it was to be used. Thin slices (3–4 mm) were fixed either 4–5 h at 25°C or 24 h at 4°C. It has previously been reported from this laboratory that Carnoy's fluid does not alter significantly the susceptibility or resistance of connective tissue macromolecules and macromelecular complexes to enzymatic digestions and chemical extractions[20]. Other authors emphasized that after Carnoy's fixation optimal results can be obtained concerning the action of collagenase on collagen fibers[21]. Fixation in Carnoy's fluid also enabled satisfactory preservation of macromolecular complexes rich in acidic and alcohol groups[22–25] and was recommended for the preservation of sulfhydryls[22].

After fixation, the tissue specimens were transferred to absolute ethyl alcohol for 2–4 h, followed by an additional washing in fresh absolute ethyl alcohol for 2–4 h and were then embedded in paraffin in the usual way.

Histochemical analysis of constitutive substances

The histochemical reactivity of sialic acid was demonstrated by the staining difference with Alcian blue with and without prior sialidase digestion. For this purpose the following solutions have been used: (i) 1% Alcian blue "Erich Nickel" in 3% acetic acid at pH 2.5 for 2–3 h at 25°C. (ii) Sialidase "Wellcome" 1 ml : 4 ml of 0.2 M acetate buffer (pH 5.2) for 24 h at 37°C, control slides being placed in the buffer solution. Sections of rabbit and guinea pig salivary glands have been employed to test the ability of sialidase to digest the mucin (pH 2.5) alcianophilic material, demonstrated by chemical methods to be sialic acid[26,43]. The absence of proteolytic activity was revealed by incubation for 18–24 h at 37°C with crystalline serum albumin as substrate. After deproteinization at 40°C with trichloroacetic acid made up to 5%, the precipitate was centrifuged down and an aliquot of the supernatant was subjected to paper chromatography (Whatman No. 1 or 3) using N-butanol–acetic acid as solvent. The spots were developed with ninhydrin. The absence of spots and the absence of digestion of smears of purified hyaluronic acid and chondroitin-sulfates were considered as an additional test of sialidase specificity.

Chondroitin-sulfates A and/or C have been revealed by means of basophilic dyes used prior and after testicular hyaluronidase digestion. An enzyme supplied by Nutritional Biochemicals Corporation was used, 1 mg/ml 0.85% NaCl solution, for 24 h at 37°C, control slides being placed in physiological saline solution. The absence of proteolytic activity was controlled as well as the ability of the enzyme to digest smears of purified hyaluronic acid and chondroitin-sulfates A and/or C.

The presence of galactose was revealed by staining differences with PAS prior and after galactosidase digestion. Likewise Alcian blue staining was employed to indicate a possible removal of galactose with its bound sialic acid. A galactosidase furnished by Serva was used, 2 mg : ml McIlvain buffer (pH 6.4) for 24 h at 37°C, control slides being placed in buffer alone.

Hexosamines have been investigated by means of lysozyme digestion (β-glucosaminidase wich acts on N-acetylated glucosamines in oligosaccharides[27]), followed by PAS staining. For this purpose a lysozyme supplied by Worthington Biochemicals Corporation was used, 5 mg/30 ml 0.2 M phosphate buffer (pH 5.3) for

48 h at 37°C, control slides being placed in the buffer solution as well as in lysozyme inactivated by Lugol's iodine 1 : 300 buffer.

The presence of non-collagen proteins was demonstrated by means of tetrazotized benzidine coupled with either β-naphthol or H-acid[23]. This method shows the collective presence of histidine, tryptophan and tyrosine and thereby proteins in general. Likewise pepsin and trypsin digestions were associated, these two endopeptidases being able to hydrolyze the internal peptide bonds as well as those of the terminal amino acid of proteins[22-24]. The digestions were performed with enzymes supplied by Difco: pepsin 2 mg/ml 0.02 N HCl at pH 1.6 for 1–3 h at 37°C, control slides being placed in HCl solution; trypsin 0.1 mg/ml phosphate buffer 0.05 M (pH 8.9) for 1–3 h at 37°C, control slides being placed in phosphate buffer.

To reveal mucoprotein complexes we used papain digestion prior to toluidine blue staining, as well as prior to PAS, alcian blue and tetrazotized benzidine. The digestions were performed with papain supplied by Difco 2 g/100 ml phosphate buffer 0.06 M (pH 6.5) for 3–6 h at 52°C, control slides being incubated in buffer alone or in papain inactivated with iodoacetate 10 mg per 100 ml. The specificity of the enzyme was tested on rabbits and guinea pig cartilage.

Collagen, histologically characterized by red staining with Van Gieson picrofuchsin and turning light-brown upon silver impregnation, was identified by means of collagenase digestion; the collagenase employed in this work was supplied by Nutritional Biochemicals Corporation 1 mg/ml phosphate buffer 0.1 M (pH 7.3) for 3–24 h at 37°C, control slides being placed in buffer alone. The enzyme, purified by ion-exchange chromatography, was tested on the pig skin, the specific action being evaluated as the ability to remove the picrofuchsinophilic material of dermal collagen fibers. The same enzyme when used by other authors[28] was capable of digesting 145–150 mg of beef tendon collagen per mg of enzyme in 30 min.

Finally some bound lipids, resistant to Carnoy's fixation and embedding in paraffin, were revealed using extractions techniques (acetone, diethyl ether and equal parts chloroform and methyl alcohol, for 24 h at 25°C and 60°C) followed by staining with Sudan Black B (National Aniline No. 629) in propylene glycol[23] as well as with performic or peracetic acid-Schiff[22].

Histochemical analysis of end groups

The investigation of the reactive chemical end groups was carried out using both specific staining reactions and blockades. Evaluation of the results of blockades has been made by comparing the optical aspect of the sections stained with the specific reagent used as controls with the sections treated with the blocking agent.

Acidic groups: (i) Phosphate–HCl buffer solution of 0.05% toluidine blue Merck at a pH varying from 1.4–6.5 for 3 min at 25°C. (ii) Methylation for blocking carboxyl groups as a result of an esterification without hydrolysis and for eliminating sulfate radicals[22-24]. Demethylation was accomplished with a 1% KOH solution in 80% ethyl alcohol.

Alcohol groups: (i) PAS, performed as usual[29]. (ii) Sulfation for 12 min at 0°C

141

(ref. [30]) followed by staining with 0.05% toluidine blue (pH 2.5) for 30 min, to introduce sulfate esters due to the ability of sulfuric acid to esterify the hydroxyl groups of carbohydrates. (iii) Acetylation, to block hydroxyl radicals or aminohydroxy groups[22-24]. (iv) Phenylhydrazine both before oxidation (to block preexistent aldehydes) and afterwards (to block those formed as a result of oxidation of hydroxyl radicals)[22-24].

Amino groups: The ninhydrin and alloxan-Schiff reactions[31] were employed, associated with a Van Slyke mixture and chloramine T, to remove the amino groups[24].

Sulfhydryl groups: (i) The dihydroxynaphthyl disulfite method of BARRNETT AND SELIGMAN was utilized, its specificity being tested using the pretreatment with iodine prior to a thioglycolic acid–sodium hydroxyide bath[22,32]. (ii) Blockade was accomplished by N-ethyl-maleimide[32].

Histochemical analysis of linkages

Investigations performed in our laboratory[20,33,34] have proposed several histochemical techniques for revealing the main type of linkages which assure the strength of macromolecular aggregation. In this paper we have utilized:

(i) 0.85 and 10% NaCl (3, 6, 12, 24 and 40 h at 37°C) to disrupt electrostatic linkages, control slides being placed in distilled water. Chemical data have indicated that at low salt concentration (*e.g.* 0.15 M NaCl) only α chains of collagen macromolecules are dissolved. After increasing the salt concentration varying proportions of α and β components are broken up[35].

(ii) 8 M urea in Sörensen buffer 0.06 M (pH7.4) (3, 6, 12, and 24 h at 37°C), control slides being placed in Sörensen buffer. It is widely accepted that a tissue that is stabilized by intermolecular hydrogen bonds can be disrupted by unbond ions which compete with electrical charges forming the hydrogen bonds[36]. In this respect, a powerful hydrogen-bonding agent, such as urea, affects macromolecules by competing for hydrogen bonding sites. Studies with polarized light have demonstrated that hydrogen bridges, which urea destroys, are important factors in stabilizing collagen fibers[37].

(iii) 1% KOH in 80% ethanol (3, 6, 12 and 24 h at 37°C), control slides being placed in 80% ethanol. Alkali extraction is widely used, the sensitivity of glycosidic bonds to dilute alkali being repeatedly emphasized[38]. Destruction of serine, concomitant with the separation of protein and carbohydrate by mild alkaline hydrolysis (0.45 N KOH or 0.50 M NaOH), was the first concrete evidence that the hydroxyl group of serine is involved in the linkage between acid mucopolysaccharides and proteins[39].

The prevalence of a certain type of linkage in each macromolecular complex and in each age group was demonstrated by staining differences with toluidine blue, alcian blue, PAS, Gomori's silver impregnation, Van Gieson's picrofuchsin, Weigert's resorcin–fuchsin, with and without prior 0.85 and 10% NaCl, 8 M urea and 1% KOH extractions.

RESULTS

0–7-year-old group

The results are based only on lesion-free specimens obtained until 6–8 h post mortem.

Histological aspects. In serial sections, in 31 out of 60 specimens (more than 50%), a minimal thickening was encountered in the intima of the cerebral arteries. It was related topographically to the splitting, reduplication and/or fragmentation of the internal elastic membrane, occurring as a narrow subendothelial concentration of a toluidine blue metachromatic material, in which silver impregnation techniques revealed a few reticular networks randomly oriented. Collagen and elastic fibers were absent. This histological aspect permitted differentiation of the occasional intimal thickening from the normal pads and cushions which exist at particular anatomical sites of branching. In these pads and cushions well-developed elastic, collagen and

TABLE 1

MEAN VALUE OF THE INTIMA THICKENING IN THE CEREBRAL ARTERIES OF 0–7-YEAR-OLD GROUP

No. of the specimen	Age of the subject	Cause of death	Cerebral arteries	Intimal thickening (μ)
35/1	28 days	bronchopneumonia	basilar	76
35/2			vertebral	38
72/1	6 months	bronchopneumonia	basilar	82
72/2			vertebral	47
12/1	3 years	septicemia	basilar	92
12/2			vertebral	61
12/5			posterior	32
14/1	3.5 years	septicemia	basilar	78
14/2			vertebral	39
19/1	5 years	accident	basilar	182
19/2			vertebral	93
19/4			middle	65
19/5			posterior	72
48/1	6 years	septicemia	basilar	151
48/2			vertebral	94
48/4			middle	37
48/5			posterior	42
62/1	7 years	accident	basilar	153
62/2			vertebral	101
62/4			middle	72
62/5			posterior	76
66/1	7 years	encephalitis	basilar	185
66/2			vertebral	93
66/3			anterior	46
66/4			middle	52
66/5			posterior	83
67/1	7 years	peritonitis	basilar	174
67/2			vertebral	96
67/3			anterior	33
67/4			middle	53
67/5			posterior	78

reticular fibers occur, circularly disposed, displaying a particular concentric orientation in parallel layers.

The minimal intimal thickening encountered in our material exhibited neither the aspect of a clearly distinct area between the endothelial cells and the media nor the aspect of a circumferential development of the intimal connective tissue over the whole length of the section.

In each specimen analyzed, the area of intimal thickening was measured in 5 different points with a micrometric objective. The mean values obtained are shown in Table 1. Statistical treatment of these mean values by the significance test of the difference between means (t test) revealed, in each particular subject, a highly significant difference ($P < 0.01$) between the intimal thickening of the basilar artery, on the one hand, and that of the vertebral, anterior cerebral, middle cerebral and posterior cerebral arteries, on the other hand.

Histochemical findings. The following constitutive substances, reactive groups and types of linkages have been revealed in the macromolecular complexes which form the intimal thickening of intracranial cerebral arteries:

Chondroitin-sulfates A and/or C, demonstrated by staining differences with toluidine blue prior to and after testicular hyaluronidase digestion. Except for a narrow subendothelial zone which persisted (heparin-like substances?), the rest of the toluidine blue metachromatic material disappeared subsequent to hyaluronidase incubation.

Sialic acid, demonstrated by staining differences with alcian blue prior to and after sialidase digestion, the enzymatic action being followed by a total removal of the alcianophilic material.

Hexoses and hexosamines, demonstrated by a decrease in the PAS affinity following galactosidase and lysozyme digestions, respectively.

Mucoproteins, a toluidine blue metachromatic material which was completely eliminated after 1–2 h of papain digestion.

Non-collagen proteins, a substrate stained with tetrazotized benzidine coupled with either β-naphthol or H-acid and susceptible to pepsin and trypsin digestions.

Acidic groups, especially related to the presence of sialic acid, stainable starting from a pH 2.2, a fully developed metachromasia being observed at pH 3.6. These acidic functions appeared totally deblocked after methylation and saponification, indicating the prevalence of carboxyl radicals.

Alcohol groups, especially of vic-glycol type, belonging to hexoses an hexosamines (also fucose?), occurring completely blocked after acetylation and deblocked following saponification.

Amino groups and sulfhydryl groups, showing a weak histochemical reactivity.

Extraction with 0.85% and 10% NaCl was followed by a total dissolution of the toluidine blue metachromatic material, suggesting the prevalence of electrostatic bonds between macromolecules of mucoprotein complexes. On the contrary, sialoproteins and glycoproteins (or sialoglycoproteins) persisted after the same pretreatment. After 1% KOH extraction, both toluidine blue and PAS reactive substrata have been eliminated.

Conclusion: the intimal connective tissue of cerebral arteries of the 0–7-year-old group is formed by macromolecular complexes including: sialic acid, chondroitin-sulfates A and/or C, hexoses, hexosamines, non-collagen proteins. These substances occur as mucoprotein, glycoprotein or sialoglycoprotein complexes, displaying a histochemical prevalence of carboxyl and vic-glycol groups, as well as a histochemical prevalence of electrostatic linkages in the mucoprotein complexes and of covalent linkages in the glycoprotein complexes. Our methods did not enable demonstration of any heparin-like substances, fucose, elastin and collagen macromolecules non-integrated in fibrillar structures.

21–42-year-old group

The results are based only on lesion-free specimens obtained until 6–8 h post mortem.

Histological aspects. The intimal thickening was constantly encountered, at least focally, in every sample examined on serial sections. Our data concerning the intimal thickening in this group are superposable in relation to those published by other authors on 30–39-year-old subjects[19].

In 15 samples (25%), this intimal thickening apparently developed over the whole length of the section, irrespective of the degree of light microscopic alterations (on conventional techniques) of the internal elastic lamellae.

The most important histological observation noted in this group is the progressive transformation of the intimal connective tissue. In this newly formed layer, it was possible to visualize in young adults delicate elastic fibers and membranes, intermingled with a few fuchsinophilic collagen fibers, with an intense argyrophilic reticular network and with an abundant metachromatic ground substance. Except for smooth muscle cells, irregularly arranged, only occasional histocytes and fibroblasts were encountered. However, in several sections, the smooth muscle cells of the intima were sometimes small, delicate and difficult to recognize as such by the light microscope. This apparently homogeneous aspect of the intimal connective tissue was progressively replaced by a heterogeneous aspect, characterized by the differentiation of two sublayers, an inner, juxtaluminal and an outer, juxtamedial sublayer. The process of intimal subdivision developed very slowly and began to be visualized when the intimal thickness had reached more than 300 μ, as can be seen in Fig. 1.

The inner, juxtaluminal sublayer was poor in ground substance, elastic fibers and collagen fibers, but exhibited a well-developed reticular network. It displayed the general aspect of the loose fibrillar connective tissue. The outer, juxtamedial sublayer occurred as a dense connective tissue with a dense accumulation of reticular, elastic and collagen fibers.

Histochemical findings. The above-mentioned histological changes were accompanied by the following modifications of the histochemical pattern of the young group:

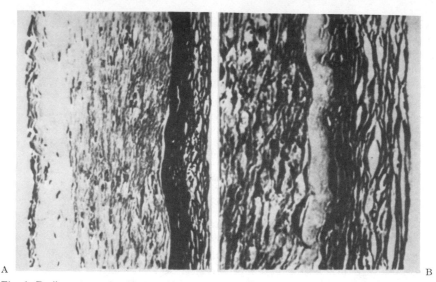

A   B

Fig. 1. Basilar artery of a 42-year-old subject. *A*: Differentiation in the newly formed intimal connective tissue of two sublayers: an inner, juxtaluminal intimal sublayer displaying a loose fibrillar structure and an outer, juxtamedial intimal sublayer composed of a denser connective tissue. Toluidine blue, pH 5.0. × 220. *B*: Colloidal iron technique, permitting delineation of the topographical relationship between the outer intimal sublayer and the internal elastic membrane. × 440.

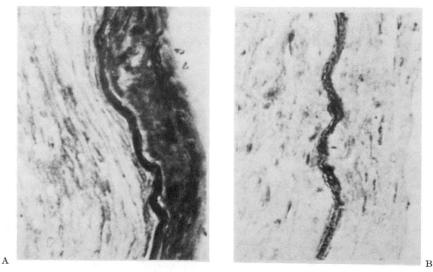

A   B

Fig. 2. Vertebral artery of a 22-year-old subject. *A*: Intense metachromasia of the newly formed intimal connective tissue. *B*: Disappearance of the metachromatic substrate after sialidase digestion. Toluidine blue, pH 5.0 × 440.

146

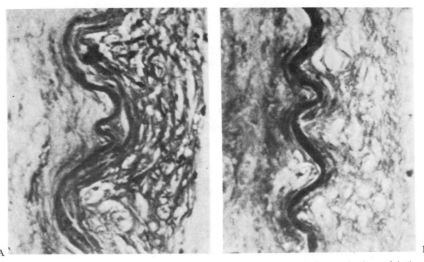

A

B

Fig. 3. Vertebral artery of a 46-year-old subject. *A*: Persistence of the newly formed intimal connective tissue metachromasia, after sialidase digestion. *B*: Disappearance of the metachromatic material following 1% KOH pretreatment and sialidase digestion. Toluidine blue, pH 5.0. × 440.

A progressive increase in the resistance of chondroitin-sulfate A and/or C, sialic acid, mucoproteins and non-collagen proteins to the specific enzymatic digestion. For instance, in some samples from subjects aged 21–25 years, the same susceptibility to sialidase was noted as in the young group (Fig. 2). On the contrary, in samples belonging to subjects aged 40–42 years, there was either no digestion or only partial digestion. The same aspects were encountered subsequent to testicular hyaluronidase incubation. Short proteolytic digestions with pepsin or trypsin and especially a brief pretreatment with 1% KOH rendered the metachromatic and alcianophilic substrate again susceptible to the above-mentioned enzymes. The effect of 1% KOH occurred as very important for the removal of sialic acid subsequent to sialidase digestion (Fig. 3). Papain was unable to degrade mucoproteins in 1–2 h as in the young group, 3–4 h being necessary for the adult one. Likewise, non-collagen proteins were hydrolyzed in about 30 min by pepsin and trypsin in the young group, requiring more than 1 h in the adult one. On the contrary, the PAS-reactive material exhibited an apparently similar susceptibility to galactosidase and lysozyme incubations. As concerns the newly formed collagen fibers occurring as a fuchsinophilic material, they disappeared constantly after 3 h of collagenase digestion.

A decrease in the intimal isoelectric point, but only in 21–25-year-old subjects (basophilia starting from pH 1.8, a fully developed metachromasia at pH 3.2), followed by an increase of the isoelectric point till 3.2 in the mature adults, 38–42 years of age (basophilia starting from pH 3.2, a fully developed metachromasia at pH 4.4). The young adults exhibited an important loss of acidic functions following methylation-

147

saponification, whereas the mature adults showed an unaltered pattern of meta-chromasia.

An important increase in the histochemical reactivity of the amino groups took place in adults, especially in the outer intimal sublayer.

Extractions with 0.85% and 10% NaCl or with 8 M urea were followed by only a partial degradation of the mucoproteins, suggesting a progressive increase in covalent linkages between macromolecules. This assumption was supported by the persistence of the susceptibility to 1% KOH extraction. Glycoproteins resisted all bond-breaking agents used in this work, whereas the newly formed collagen fibers were dissolved in physiological saline solution and urea.

Conclusions: The intimal connective tissue of the adult cerebral arteries exhibited an increase in the strength of linkages between various types of macromolecules and macromolecular complexes, leading to a limitation of enzyme–substrate interaction, as well as to an augmented resistance to various bond-breaking agents. Likewise a partial blockade of the sulfate groups by basic proteins occurred.

62–78-year-old group

The material utilized included both specimens without lesions and specimens with early atheromatous alterations.

Histological aspects. Data concerning the intimal thickening are comparable with those published by other authors concerning a 60–69-year-old group[19].

In older age groups the diffuse intimal thickening varied considerably from case

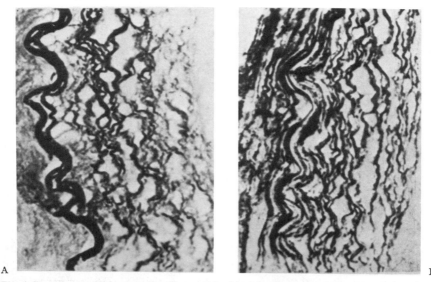

A   B

Fig. 4. Posterior cerebral artery of a 68-year-old subject. Progressive and spontaneous disappearance, in the inner, juxtaluminal intimal sublayer, of elastic (*A*) and reticular (*B*) fibres. *A*: Weigert's resorcin-fuchsin, *B*: Gomori's silver impregnation. × 440.

148

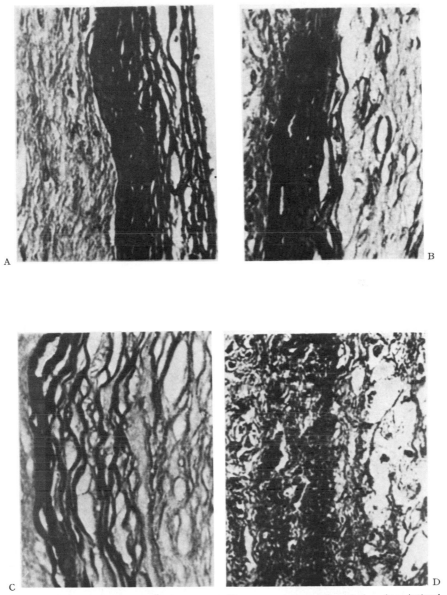

Fig. 5. Basilar artery of a 68-year-old subject. *A*: The same aspect of differentiation of two intimal sublayers as in Fig. 1A. *B*: Adjacent area, exhibiting a transformation of the inner, juxtaluminal intimal sublayer into a mucoid-edematous tissue. Toluidine blue, pH 5.0. *C*: Accumulation of elastic lamellae and fibers in the juxtamedial sublayer, associated with the disappearance of elastic tissue in the juxtaluminal sublayer displaying the aspect of mucoid tissue. Weigert's resorcin–fuchsin, × 440. *D*: Transformation of the mucoid tissue into an atheroma plaque. The juxtamedial sublayer occurs as a hyalinized band of connective tissue. Hematoxylin–eosin. × 440.

to case, as did the alterations of the internal elastic membrane. It is important to note that this group did not exhibit an intima with an increasingly fibrous character and that real scar formation was not encountered.

The separation of the intimal connective tissue into two sublayers appeared more prominent as in the adult group. In addition, a particular transformation in the inner, juxtaluminal sublayer occurred, some limited areas of about 1 mm displaying the aspect of a loose-mucoid and edematous tissue. In these regions elastic fibers were split into a less dense material or exhibited striking discontinuities, small fragments or granular deposits in place of preexisting "normal" histologic structures (Fig. 4A). Likewise a spontaneous dissolution of reticular (Fig. 4B) and collagen fibers was noted. These limited areas of mucoid degeneration were more frequently encountered in basilar arteries than in vertebral ones, and more in vertebral than in middle and posterior cerebral arteries. Fig. 5 illustrates the transformation of some regions of the inner, juxtaluminal intimal sublayer, from a loose fibrillar connective tissue into an edematous loose-mucoid area and then into an atheroma plaque. In the same figure is illustrated the accumulation of elastic, collagen and reticular fibers in the juxtamedial intimal sublayer, exhibiting a definite parallel orientation to the internal elastic membrane. No calcification or lipid deposits were encountered in this sublayer, which seems to form a mechanical barrier which blocks lipid accumulation in the juxtaluminal intimal sublayer, as it can been seen in Fig. 5D. The fibers of the juxtamedial sublayer often seemed to coalesce and to stain variable with eosin and appeared as if they had become "hyalinized" (Figs. 5B and D). Some reticular and elastic fibers also

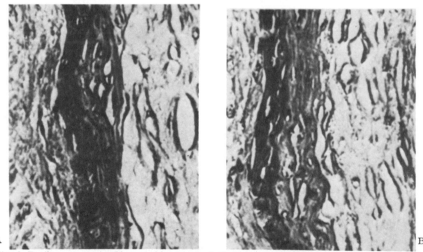

Fig. 6. Basilar artery of a 72-year-old subject. *A*: Section submitted to successive trypsin (1 h), 1 % KOH (30 min) and sialidase (24 h) treatments. The metachromatic substrate of the outer intimal sublayer persisted. *B*: Adjacent section submitted to successive trypsin, 1 % KOH and testicular hyaluronidase (24 h) treatments. The metachromatic material of the outer intimal sublayer persisted. Toluidine blue. × 440.

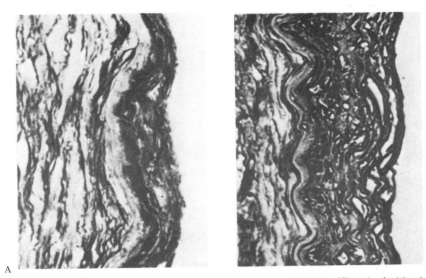

A   B

Fig. 7. Vertebral artery of a 7-year-old subject (*A*) and 74-year-old subject (*B*) stained with tolui dine blue, pH 4.4. *A*: Intense metachromasia of the newly formed intimal connective tissue. *B*: Slight metachromasia of the newly formed intimal connective tissue, especially in the inner intimal sublayer. × 440.

became fuchsinophilic. Such "collagenization" of non-collagen fibers can be consider- ed a prominent feature of the aged cerebral arteries. On the contrary, no significant coarsening and thickening of the "true" collagen fibers was observed in our material.

Histochemical findings. In the outer, juxtamedial intimal sublayer, the resistance of chondroitin-sulfate A and/or C, sialic acid, mucoproteins and non-collagen proteins to enzymatic digestions was more prominent than in the adult group. Likewise such substances as hexoses, hexosamines and collagen, removed in the adult group follow- ing galactosidase, lysozyme and collagenase incubations, respectively, also became resistant to the action of the specific ferments. Short proteolytic pretreatments with pepsin and trypsin as well as with 1 % KOH were unable to restore the initial sus- ceptibility to enzymatic digestions of chondroitin-sulfates and sialic acid (Fig. 6).

The isoelectric point of the same outer, juxtamedial intimal sublayer rose from pH 3.2 in the adult group to a pH of 4.0 (Fig. 7), a complete metachromasia develop- ing only starting from pH 5.0. Methylation, followed by saponification, restored with more intensity the initial toluidine blue metachromasia.

The blockade following acetylation and the subsequent saponification were followed only by a partial reactivity of the PAS-positive material, suggesting a partici- pation of proteins in the PAS affinity of the outer medial sublayer. The techniques of staining non-collagen proteins produced more intense results than in the adult group. Likewise collagen fibers exhibited a more prominent affinity for Van Gieson's picro- fuchsin and in some cases were also PAS-reactive, displaying the aspect of "hyalinized" structures.

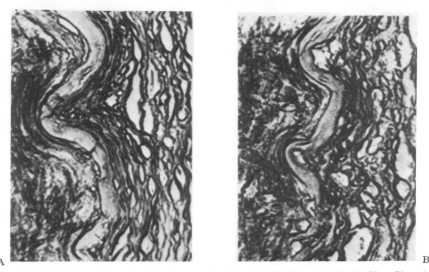

A   B

Fig. 8. Posterior cerebral artery of a 66-year-old subject. *A*: Section stained with Van Gieson's picrofuchsin. *B*: Section submitted to 8 *M* urea for 24 h at 37 °C and then stained with Van Gieson's picrofuchsin. Persistence of the fuchsinophilic material in the outer, juxtamedial intimal sublayer. × 440.

As judged by the eye, extractions with 0.85% and 10% NaCl, 8 *M* urea and 1% KOH did not significantly alter the staining affinities for toluidine blue, alcian blue, PAS, ammoniacal silver solution and Van Gieson's picrofuchsin in the outer, juxtamedial intimal sublayer (Fig. 8).

In the inner, juxtaluminal intimal sublayer, a prevalence of degenerative processes occurred. Consequently, a progressive dissolution of the ground substance was noted, leading to a progressive diminution of metachromasia. The remaining macromolecular complexes appeared only with a β-metachromasia, similar to that encountered in myxedema. The reticular fibers exhibited a loosening of their intermolecular bonds, being dissolved after a pretreatment with an electrostatic bond breaker, such as 10% NaCl. The mechanism of elastic and collagen fiber dissolution requires complementary studies.

Conclusion: The intimal connective tissue of the 62–78-year-old group exhibits a progressive amplification of the age-related changes mentioned in the adult group. In the outer, juxtamedial intimal sublayer abnormal macromolecular complexes are formed, resistant to enzymatic digestions and chemical extractions. On the contrary, in the inner, juxtaluminal intimal sublayer a prevalence of degenerative processes was encountered which seems to favor the development of atherosclerotic lesions.

The particular type of macromolecular composition, organization and aggregation occurring in the two intimal sublayers in the older age group could not be correlated in our material with the mean thickness of the respective intima, by the ratio intima/media, by the ratio intima/arterial wall, or by the alterations of the internal elastic membrane visualized by means of conventional methods.

The main demonstrative results obtained in our histochemical analysis of various age groups are presented in Tables 2–4.

DISCUSSION

The purpose of the current investigation was to study histologically and histo-chemically some age-related changes occurring in the cerebral arteries, in order to emphasize their significance in the development of atherosclerosis.

The exact nature of numerous histochemical reactions presented in this paper are not fully understood and cannot be equated in detail with chemical formulae. However, despite these limitations, our results strongly suggest that the intimal connective tissue of the cerebral arteries undergoes spontaneous qualitative and quantitative modifications during the course of aging. This often-ignored phenomenon of macromolecules and macromolecular complexes *in vivo* is reflected *in vitro* by a modified histochemical pattern concerning: chemical components, reactive groups, electrical charge, susceptibility to enzymatic digestions, resistance to chemical ex-tractions, etc.

The occurrence of similar age-related changes in adults and the older age group

TABLE 2

CEREBRAL ARTERIES. RELATIONSHIP BETWEEN AGING AND ENZYMATIC SUSCEPTIBILITY OF SOME COMPONENTS OF THE INTIMAL CONNECTIVE TISSUE

Substance	0–7–year-old group	21–42-year-old group	62–78-year-old group
Sialic acid			
sialidase 24 h	digested	partly digested	not digested
KOH + sialidase	digested	digested	partly digested
			not digested
Chondroitin-sulfates			
testic.hyaluron. 24 h	digested	partly digested	not digested
trypsin + testic. hyal.	digested	digested	partly digested
			not digested
Hexoses			
galactosidase 24 h	partly digested	partly digested	not digested
Hexosamines			
lysozyme 48 h	partly digested	partly digested	not digested
Mucoproteins			
papain 2 h	digested	partly digested	not digested
papain 6 h	digested	digested	partly digested
Non-collagen proteins			
trypsin 30 min	digested	partly digested	not digested
trypsin 2 h	digested	digested	partly digested
			not digested
Collagen			
collagenase 3 h	not done	digested	not digested
collagenase 12 h	not done	digested	partly digested
			not digested

TABLE 3

CEREBRAL ARTERIES. RELATIONSHIP BETWEEN AGING AND HISTOCHEMICAL REACTIVITY OF VARIOUS RADICALS

Chemical radicals	0–7-year-old group	21–42-year-old group	62–78-year-old group
Acidic functions (sialic acid and acid mucopolysaccharides)			
carboxyl	moderate	moderate	intense
sulfate	weak	moderate (young adults) weak (mature adults)	weak
blockade following methylation and saponification:	absent	partial (young adults) absent (mature adults)	absent
basophilia pH	2.2	1.8–3.2	4.0
metachromasia pH	3.6	3.2–4.4	5.0
Alcohol functions (sialoglycoproteins)			
vic-glycols	moderate	moderate (subluminal) intense (juxtamedial)	weak (subluminal) intense (juxtamedial)
hydoxyls: sulfation	weak moderate	weak moderate	weak
Amino (proteins)	weak	weak moderate	moderate (juxtamedial)
Sulfhydryls (proteins)	weak	weak moderate	moderate (juxtamedial)

with both "normal" and atherosclerotic cerebral arteries suggests that the passage of plasma constituents through the vessel wall exhibiting an altered pattern of macromolecular organization and aggregation is not the unique factor which determines the onset of lesions. Consequently some "local" haemodynamic and metabolic conditions must be taken into consideration in the pathogenesis of the disease.

One of the most prominent and constant changes encountered in our material was the progressive blockade of acidic functions by basic proteins, starting from the 4th decade of life. It is generally accepted that acid mucopolysaccharides are macromolecules of a strong polyelectrolyte character, acting *in vivo* as a cation-exchange resin[40]. In this respect excellent correlations have been noted between the cation-binding capacity of acid mucopolysaccharides and their sulfate content[41]. Studies on the change in connective tissue colloidal charge density with atherosclerosis and age pointed out that the greater charge density might be associated with a greater resistance to atherosclerosis[42]. Thus it is tempting to assume that the spontaneous decrease with aging in the charge density of the intimal connective tissue of the cerebral arteries might lead to alterations of intimal permeability, of the microenvironment of the intima and even of the local cellular metabolism.

TABLE 4

CEREBRAL ARTERIES. RELATIONSHIP BETWEEN AGING AND RESISTANCE TO CHEMICAL PROCEDURES
OF INTIMAL MACROMOLECULES

Methods	0–7-year-old group	21–42-year-old group	62–78-year-old group
0.85% NaCl			
mucoproteins	extracted	partly extracted	not extracted
glycoproteins	not extracted	not extracted	not extracted
reticular fibers	not extracted	not extracted	partly extracted
collagen fibers	not done	extracted	not extracted
10% NaCl			
mucoproteins	extracted	partly extracted	not extracted
glycoproteins	not extracted	not extracted	not extracted
reticular fibers	not extracted	not extracted	partly extracted
collagen fibers	not done	extracted	not extracted
8 M urea			
mucoproteins	extracted	partly extracted	not extracted
glycoproteins	not extracted	not extracted	not extracted
reticular fibers	not extracted	not extracted	not extracted
collagen fibers	not done	extracted	not extracted
1% KOH			
mucoproteins	extracted	extracted	partly extracted
glycoproteins	partly extracted	not extracted	not extracted
reticular fibers	not extracted	not extracted	partly extracted
collagen fibers	not done	extracted	not extracted

A second important change was the progressive lack of susceptibility to enzymatic digestions of sialic acid, chondroitin-sulfates, hexoses, hexosamines, mucoproteins, non-collagen proteins, and collagen fibers. This resistance reflects a different steane configuration, less susceptible to the specific requirements of each enzyme, and might be due: (i) to the mode of attachment; (ii) to a change bond configuration; (iii) to a change residue to which the respective substance was attached. For instance, sialic acid has usually been found linked cetosidically to galactose or N-acetyl-galactosamine, the sialidase-susceptible bond having a configuration[43]. The occurrence of O-acetyl substitute (O-acetylgalactosamine) has been reported to be responsible for the resistance of sialic acid to sialidase. This resistance can be eliminated after 1% KOH pretreatment, subsequent to hydrolysis of the O-acetyl group, since such an ester bond is alkali labile[44]. Correlating these findings with our results, an assumption can be made that in the mature adults and older age subjects a progressive substitution of N-acetyl by O-acetyl occurs in the preterminal carbohydrate fraction of the oligosaccharide chain of the intimal connective tissue glycoproteins. Unfortunately the specific functional significance of this change is still conjectural.

A third important change is, in our opinion, the continuous modifications in the abundance, type and distribution of inter- and intramolecular bonds, leading to the appearance of the dense connective tissue in the juxtamedial intimal sublayer, displaying features of "hyalinization" and "collagenization" of numerous structures. It represents, probably, an inadequate repair reaction to compensate, functionally, for the changes in the internal elastic membrane, although it may help to reenforce the arterial wall. It was postulated that the age-dependent cross-linkages in aortic wall protein chains is manifested essentially by changes in the mechanical and surface properties of the intima and in the transintimal passage of blood constituents[45]. The abnormal development of linkages in the outer intimal sublayer could help to explain the progressive decrease in distensibility and the increase in the rate of change in slope (or the curvature) of pressure–volumes curves toward the pressure axis[46], revealed in aging arteries. The occurrence of these abnormal macromolecular complexes, including also collagen and elastic fibers, alters the functional capacity of the collagen–elastic system to act as a "two-phase" material, such as fiberglass[47]. Consequently, an inadequate modification in the ability of cerebral arteries to adjust to changing demands might occur and this altered nutrition of the arterial wall could explain: the increase in intimal permeability, the state of edema, the stagnation of blood constituents and the spontaneous degeneration of reticular, elastic and collagen fibers.

In the cerebral arteries it was not possible to demonstrate that the high frequency of atherosclerosis in older age is primarily due to an increase in the intimal thickness, as in the coronary arteries[19]. Our results reenforce this conclusion, suggesting that β-lipoproteins and fibrinogen are not trapped as a result of an increased filtration "distance" between the endothelium and the media but probably as a result of a mechanical barrier formed by the abnormal macromolecular complexes of the outer intimal sublayer.

Unfortunately, no relation can be made between our qualitative findings, based on histochemical methods alone, and quantitative chemical estimations. There are no published data in the available literature on the chemistry of cerebral arteries related to the process of aging, and it is not adequate to apply to this particular vascular area the results obtained in the chemical analysis of aortic acid mucopolysaccharides, glycoproteins, non-collagen proteins, collagen and elastin macromolecules. We hope that our modest contribution will serve to stimulate such chemical investigations, as did some previous publications which emphasized:

The presence in the cerebral arteries of a thicker and denser internal elastic membrane than in other vascular beds[48,49]; the occurrence in the cerebral arteries of senescent individuals of a less frequent and less severe calcification than in coronary arteries[19,50]; the existence in the cerebral arteries of a significantly lower content of hexosamine, uronic acid and sulfur than that in other arteries[51], associated with both a chemical[51] and a histochemical[16] absence of hyaluronic acid; the ability of the cerebral arteries to metabolize lipids in a different fashion than do coronary arteries, with less accumulation of a cholesterol ester[19].

REFERENCES

1 KURTZKE, J. F., *Epidemiology of Cerebrovascular Diseases*, Springer, Berlin, 1969, p. 124.
2 TICHY, J., H. SVABOVE-TICHE AND V. MALY, Cancer in relation to diseases with disorders of cholesterol metabolism, *Cas. Lék. Cés.*, 1953, 92: 1004.

[3] WINTER, M. D., JR., G. P. SAYER, C. H. MILLIKAN AND N. W. BARKER, Relationship of degree of atherosclerosis of internal carotid system in the brain of women to age and coronary atherosclerosis, *Circulation*, 1958, 18: 7.

[4] MOOSY, J., Development of cerebral atherosclerosis in various age groups, *Neurology*, 1959, 9: 569.

[5] GIERSTON, J. C., Atherosclerosis in an autopsy series, Part 3 (Interrelationship between atherosclerosis in the aorta, in the coronary bed and in the cerebral arteries), *Acta Pathol. Microbiol. Scand.*, 1964, 63: 391.

[6] JEAGERMAN, K. AND PRÓCHNICKA, Variations in the occurrence and intensity of atherosclerosis in the main arterial regions, *Acta Med. Pol.*, 1965, 6: 473.

[7] ADAMS, C. W. M., *Vascular Histochemistry*, Lloyd–Luke, London, 1967, p. 15.

[8] TOOLE, J. F. AND A. N. PATEL, *Cerebrovascular Disorders*, McGraw–Hill, New York, 1967, p. 7.

[9] FLORA, G. C., A. B. BAKER AND A. KLASSEN, Age and cerebral atherosclerosis, *J. Neurol. Sci.*, 1968, 6: 357.

[10] HAKEL, W. M., Anatomy of the blood supply to the brain and senile changes, *Virchows Arch. Pathol. Anat.*, 1928, 266: 630.

[11] WOLKOFF, K., Normal structure and age-changes of the cerebral arteries, *Beitr. pathol. Anat. Allgem. Pathol.*, 1933, 91: 51.

[12] BAKER, A. B., Structure of the small cerebral arteries and their changes with age, *Am. J. Pathol.*, 1937, 13: 453.

[13] FORBUS, W. D., On the origin of milliary aneurysm of the superficial cerebral arteries, *Bull. Johns Hopkins Hosp.*, 1930, 47: 239.

[14] GLYNN, L. E., Medial defects in the circle of Willis and their relation to aneurysm formation, *J. Pathol. Bacteriol.*, 1940, 51: 213.

[15] CARMICHAEL, R., Gross defects in the muscular and elastic coats of the larger cerebral arteries, *J. Pathol. Bacteriol.*, 1945, 57: 345.

[16] ZUGIBE, F. T., The demonstration of the individual acid mucopolysaccharides in human aorta, coronary arteries and cerebral arteries, Part 2 (Identification and significance with aging), *J. Histochem. Cytochem.*, 1962, 10: 448.

[17] ZUGIBE, F. T. AND K. D. BROWN, Histochemistry of cerebral arteries, *Circulation*, 1959, 20: 971.

[18] ZUGIBE, F. T. AND K. D. BROWN, Histochemical studies in atherogenesis. Human cerebral arteries, *Circulation Res.*, 1961, 9: 897.

[19] SCOTT, R. F., A. S. DAOUD, B. WORTMAN, E. S. MORRISON AND J. JARMOLYCH, Proliferation and necrosis in coronary and cerebral arteries, *J. Atheroscler. Res.*, 1966, 6: 499.

[20] VELICAN, C. AND D. VELICAN, *Histochimie des Glucides en Pathologie Humaine*, Gauthier–Villars, Paris, 1969, p. 157.

[21] GREEN, J. A., Digestion of collagen and reticulin in paraffin sections by collagenase, *Stain Technol.*, 1960, 35: 373.

[22] LILLIE, R. D., *Histopathologic Technic and Practical Histochemistry*, 3rd Ed., McGraw–Hill, New York, N.Y., 1965.

[23] THOMPSON, S. W., *Selected Histochemical and Histopathological Methods*, Thomas, Springfield, Ill., 1966.

[24] PEARSE, A. G. E., *Histochemistry, Theoretical and Applied*, 3rd edition, Churchill, London, 1968.

[25] JÓZSA, L. AND G. SZEDERKÉNYI, Über Verluste der Gewebs-Mukopolysaccharide während der Fixierung, *Acta Histochem.*, 1967, 26: 255.

[26] SPICER, S. S. AND J. G. HENSON, Method for localizing mucosubstances in epithelial and connective tissues. In: E. BAJUSZ AND G. JASMIN (Eds.), *Methods in Achievement of Experimental Pathology*, Vol. 2, Karger, Basle, 1967, p. 78.

[27] SNELLMAN, O., A glycoprotein from reticulin tissue, *Acta Chem. Scand.*, 1963, 17: 1049.

[28] FRITZPATRICK, M. AND V. D. HOSPELHORN, Studies on human pulmonary connective tissue, Part 3 (Amino acid composition of residues following collagenase digestion of lung connective tissue), *Am. Rev. Respirat. Diseases*, 1965, 92: 792.

[29] MOWRY, R. W., The special value of methods that color both acidic and vicinal hydroxyl groups in the histochemical study of mucins, *Ann. New York Acad. Sci.*, 1963, 106: 402.

[30] MOORE, R. D. AND M. D. SCHOENBERG, Low temperature sulfation of tissues and the demonstration of metachromasy, *Stain Technol.*, 1957, 32: 245.

[31] YASUMA, A. AND T. ICHIKAWA, Ninhydrin-Schiff and alloxan-Schiff staining, *J. Lab. Clin. Med.*, 1953, 41: 269.

[32] BARRNETT, R. J. AND A. M. SELIGMAN, Histochemical demonstration of sulfhydryl and disulfide groups of proteins, *J. Natl. Cancer Inst.*, 1954, 14: 769.

[33] VELICAN, C., Histochemical analysis of the structural stability of biopolymers. Preliminary data, *Acta Histochem.*, 1968, 31: 261.

[34] VELICAN, C., Relationship between regional aortic susceptibility to atherosclerosis and macromolecular structural stability, *J. Atheroscler. Res.*, 1969, 9: 193.

157

35 BACKERMAN, S. AND R. T. HERSH, Extraction from human skin of soluble collagen molecules containing only beta components, *Nature*, 1964, **201**: 190.

36 KAHN, L. D. R., R. J. CAROLL AND L. P. WITNAUER, Some effects of electrolytes on collagen solutions, *Biochim. Biophys. Acta*, 1962, **63**: 243.

37 NEUMARK, T., Submicroscopic changes in collagen fibers of epiphyseal cartilage caused by concentrated urea, *Acta Morphol. Acad. Sci. Hung.*, 1964, **12**: 367.

38 GRANT, P. T. AND J. L. SIMKIN, Structure and biosynthesis of carbohydrate-polypeptide polymers, *J. Am. Chem. Soc.*, 1964, **61**: 491.

39 ANDERSON, B., P. HOFFMAN AND K. MEYER, A serine-linked peptide of chondroitin-sulphate, *Biochim. Biophys. Acta*, 1963, **74**: 309.

40 MEYER, K. AND M. RAPPORT, The mucopolysaccharides of the ground substance of connective tissue, *Science*, 1951, **113**: 596.

41 BOYD, E. S. AND W. F. NEUMAN, The surface chemistry of bone, *J. Biol. Chem.*, 1951, **193**: 243.

42 PORTERFIELD, S. P., T. B. CALHOON AND H. S. WEISS, Changes in connective tissue colloidal charge density with atherosclerosis and age, *Am. J. Physiol.*, 1968, **215**: 324.

43 GOTTSCHALK, A., *The Chemistry and Biology of Sialic Acid*, Cambridge University Press, London, 1960, p. 87.

44 GIBBONS, R. A., The sensitivity of the neuraminic linkage in muco-substances toward acid and toward sialidase, *Biochem. J.*, 1963, **89**: 380.

45 MILCH, R. A., J. R. JUDE AND J. KNAACK, Effects of collagen-reactive aldehyde metabolites on the structure of the canine aortic wall and their possible role in atherogenesis, *Surgery*, 1963, **54**: 104.

46 ROACH, M. R. AND C. A. BURTON, The effect of age on the elasticity of human iliac arteries, *Canad. J. Biochem.*, 1959, **37**: 577.

47 GLACOV, S. AND H. WOLINSKY, Aortic wall as a "two-phase" material, *Nature*, 1963, **199**: 606.

48 BAPTISTA, A. G., Studies on the arteries of the brain, *Angiology*, 1962, **13**: 352.

49 BLOOM, W. AND D. W. FAWCETT, *A Textbook of Histology*, Saunders, Philadelphia, London, 1962, p. 278.

50 YOUNG, W., J. W. GOFMAN, R. TANDY, N. MALAMOUD AND E. S. G. WATTER, The quantitation of atherosclerosis, Part 3 (The extent of correlation degree of atherosclerosis within and between the coronary and cerebral vascular beds), *Am. J. Cardiol.*, 1960, **6**: 300.

51 NAKAMURA, M., Y. ISHIHARA, T. SATA AND N. YABUTA, Acid mucopolysaccharides and lipids of Japanese arteries with special reference to the absence of hyaluronic acid in Japanese cerebral artery, *J. Atheroscler. Res.*, 1966, **6**: 132.

Observations on the Endothelial Nuclei of

Certain Vertebrate Extremity Veins[1]

J. KENNETH DONAHUE, ROBERT S. CONNOR AND
HAROLD W. MANNER

In his classic monograph on the veins Franklin's dictum is well taken that, "those who wish to do experimental work on any part of the venous system are well advised to study the structural peculiarities of the vein or veins upon which they propose to work" (Franklin, '37). Regarding venous endothelium in particular, the controversy among its investigators as to both its form and function could be due in part to a disregard of the significance of the location of the particular endothelium under study (Altschul, '54). The endothelium is not histologically identical in all parts of the venous system (Cunningham, '24). That it presents a smooth surface to the blood that flows within the vessel is the most obvious but certainly not the only vital function of this controversial tissue. It is also well recognized that under a variety of experimental and pathological circumstances venous endothelium is·capable of under-

[1] This investigation was supported by Public Health Service Grant 1-3573(C1) from the National Heart Institute.

going certain characteristic changes (Clark and Clark, '35; O'Neill, '47; Mehrotra, '54; Burton, '54).

The present communication is concerned with a comparative study of the endothelial nuclei of certain extremity veins in a variety of limbed vertebrates. Incidental observations on the endothelium as a whole are included with brief comments on some highly atypical conditions seen in certain extremity veins in the cow.

MATERIALS AND METHODS

Techniques have been developed by others for the study of venous endothelium but mostly in terms of the arrangement of the entire cells rather than of nuclear structure (Samuels, Samuels and Webster, '52). In an effort to determine the normal appearance of the nuclei a method was developed for studying them from their most revealing angles. In the light of the conflicting descriptions and interpretations of earlier workers it seemed imperative to standardize the preparation of tissues if the planned experimental procedures were to have an adequate basis for comparison. Representatives of several classes of vertebrate were used including the grassfrog, bullfrog, rabbit, guinea pig, dog, cow and calf. The lower femoral and tibialis veins were generally employed. To avoid post mortem distortions the veins were fixed in the living anesthetized animal (ether or Nembutal). In amphibians total immersion in a 1:1000 solution of tricaine methanesulfonate (M.S. 222)[2] gave excellent and prolonged anesthesia. The fixation procedure was standardized. Following exposure of the chosen vein, sutures were passed beneath it, one to five cm apart, and loosely tied. The fixative (Bouin's fluid or 5% glacial acetic acid in saturated corrosive sublimate) was injected into the vein with a hypodermic syringe while the blood was still flowing. The distal suture was then tied and more fixative injected into the vein in the direction of the heart. Then the proximal suture was tied. During this

[2] Courtesy of the Sandoz Chemical Company.

procedure the tissues immediately surrounding the vein were infiltrated with fixative to minimize shrinkage in the peripheral areas of the vein. The segment was then excised. Dehydration followed conventional procedures except that terpineol was used as a clearing agent. After infiltration and embedding, the sections were cut at 5 to 6 μ. In the sectioning procedure parts of the blocks were oriented to the knife so that the veins were cut along their longitudinal axis but with slight obliquity. At this angle sections were produced at the level of the endothelium which showed the nuclei almost or completely isolated from the underlying tissue and in the dimensions of their maximum length and width.

Cross sections were cut for studying the endothelial nuclei of constricted and relaxed veins as well as the remaining parts of the vein wall. Modified Harris' hematoxylin and eosin adjusted to pH 4 or Verhoeff's and Van Gieson's stain were used. The photographs were made with a Leitz Makam camera fitted with a Polaroid back.

RESULTS

Oblique sections. The photomicrographs shown in plate 1 illustrate the appearance of the endothelial nuclei of extremity veins in several species of vertebrate as seen in a plane slightly oblique to the longitudinal. It will be noted that in the 5 species represented—the grassfrog, bullfrog, dog, guinea pig, and rabbit—the morphology and cytology of the endothelial nuclei differ noticeably in detail. Standardization of the fixation procedure and the preparation of large numbers of sections from members of each species compelled the conclusion that species variations in the endothelial nuclei are not the result of the vagaries of tissue preparation.

In figures 1 and 2, the endothelial nuclei of the tibialis vein of the grassfrog (R. pipiens) are depicted. The nuclei are fusiform and show a deeply staining line running centrally from end to end.

Figure 3 shows the endothelial nuclei of the tibialis vein of the bullfrog (R. catesbiana). The nuclei are irregularly ovoid

162

in shape and contain dense, but fairly evenly dispersed, aggregations of chromatin. The dark central line seen in the grassfrog is absent in this species.

Figure 4 illustrates the endothelial nuclei in the femoral vein of the dog. The nucleus is fusiform with heavy masses of chromatin dispersed throughout.

Figure 5 shows the endothelial nuclei of the femoral vein of the guinea pig as elongated ovoid structures. The distinguishing feature of the nucleus in this species is the presence of a series of round, deeply staining chromatin bodies which stand out sharply within the nucleus and appear to be nucleoli.

Figure 6 shows the endothelial nuclei of the rabbit tibialis vein. The rabbit nucleus is a wide, ovoid structure somewhat pointed at the ends. Like that of the grassfrog, it shows a heavily staining line of chromatin along the central axis. Because of a tendency to twist, the line of chromatin occasionally appears eccentric to the central axis.

Cross sections. The ability of some veins and arteries to change their caliber to meet physiological demands is well known. This property is present in veins of the extremities and is responsible, in part at least, for the regulation of blood flowing toward the heart. In the course of this investigation the appearance of the endothelium, and particularly the endothelial nuclei, in cross sections of constricted or partially constricted veins has been noted with much interest. Conventionally the endothelium of a normal relaxed vein consists of a thin, compact cytoplasmic component containing flattened, somewhat ovate nuclei which stain heavily and uniformly with hematoxylin. However, in a state of constriction these nuclei appear swollen, assume a pear shape with the stem pointing toward the vein wall and the blunt rounded end protruding into the lumen. In this condition also the nuclear contents concentrate around the periphery leaving the central area clear. The endothelial cytoplasm becomes less compact and appears as a delicate network just below the nuclei.

163

Figure 7 depicts a conventional cross section of a relaxed femoral vein in the dog. The endothelial nuclei appear as somewhat flattened ovals when cut at this angle and lie well within the compact cytoplasm of the intima.

Figure 8 shows a cross section of a guinea pig tibialis vein in the constricted state. The swollen, pear shaped nuclei are seen protruding into the lumen. The nuclear inclusions are concentrated around the periphery of the structure leaving the center clear. The cytoplasm appears as a loose network. The long, partially constricted nucleus lying beneath the intima belongs to a smooth muscle cell in the media.

Figure 9 is a cross section of the femoral vein of a bullfrog. While the nuclei are more rounded than pear shaped, their protrusion into the lumen is clearly evident. Again the loose arrangement of the endothelial cytoplasm seen in constricted veins may be observed.

Figure 10 shows a section of a constricted tibialis vein of a pigeon, cut at a slightly oblique angle. This was selected to show the extent to which the endothelial cytoplasm sometimes expands to form a delicate network supporting the nuclei.

Figure 11 depicts a cross section of one of the lateral branches of the saphenous vein of the cow. So many atypical features were seen in bovine extremity veins that an extensive study is now being made of this species (*Bos taurus*). However, it is pertinent to this communication to point out the unusual depth of the subendothelial coat of the intima, the protrusion of the endothelial nuclei into the lumen, and the extraordinary thickness of the internal elastic layer separating the intima from the media.

In figure 12, the endothelial nuclei of a partially constricted dorsal metatarsal vein of the cow are shown ($\times$ 400). The nuclei are swollen and protrude into the lumen. The subendothelial coat of the intima is thickened but the elastic layer, seen most frequently in deeper lying veins, is absent here.

DISCUSSION

This study of the endothelial nuclei of certain extremity veins has revealed certain facts within two areas of interest. First, the study of oblique sections prepared in the manner described shows that rather marked species differences exist regarding the shape of the nucleus and the manner in which the nuclear contents are arranged. It is evident that the normal differences seen in these nuclei, from species to species, should be known by the investigator who might be studying the effects of experimental procedures upon the endothelial nuclei of the extremites.

Secondly, the response of the endothelium, including the nuclei, to venoconstriction warrants further attention in terms of its possible physiological interest. In capillaries it has been shown, for example, that in the constricted vessel the protrusion of the nuclei into the lumen serves to block the flow of blood completely (Danielli and Stock, '44). While this would not be possible in any but the smallest venules, nevertheless considerable additional diminution of lumen size would result from the protrusion of all the endothelial nuclei in a particular area of vein.

Since the authors are particularly interested in the problems of venous circulation in the so-called anti-gravity veins, the appearance of the endothelium in constricted veins, as previously described, leads us to suspect that it plays a part in the control of venous flow. Others have suggested that these changes in nuclear shape are the result of tension within the endothelial cell (Hughes, '35). There can be no doubt that a constricting venous wall would indeed effect changes in the endothelium and its nuclei. Yet, whatever the cause, an additional reduction in vein caliber results. The study of the endothelium in the living vitally stained animal utilizing the Knisely transilluminator is now in progress.

Originally, the preparation of the extremity veins of the cow for this study was done to see if conditions similar to those found in smaller vertebrates existed in this large form. As shown in plate two, the nuclei of constricted veins protrude into the lumen, but so many other atypical features were found in the vein walls in their entirety that an extensive study is being made. It may be stated here that the unusual depth of the subendothelial coat and the tortuous network of collagen and smooth muscle fibers of which it consists, may be seen consistently in the superficial veins of the lower hind leg of the cow. To our knowledge these features have never before been described.

SUMMARY

Sections cut slightly oblique to the longitudinal axis reveal the endothelial nuclei of vertebrate extremity veins relatively free of underlying tissue and in the plane of their most revealing dimensions. Species differences in the general shape of the nuclei as well as in the distribution of nuclear contents are described.

In cross sections the endothelial nuclei of constricted extremity veins appear swollen and protrude into the lumen. The endothelial cytoplasm in constricted veins loses its compact appearance and becomes a loosely arranged syncitium largely made up of collagen. The possible physiological significance of these changes is discussed.

Brief comments on the endothelial nuclei of constricted superficial extremity veins of the cow are included with remarks on some hitherto undescribed variations seen in the vein wall.

LITERATURE CITED

Altschul, R. 1954 Endothelium. The Macmillan Company, New York.

Brescher, G. A. 1956 Venous Return. Grune and Stratton, New York.

Burton, A. C. 1954 The relation of structure to function of the tissues of the walls of blood vessels. Physiol. Rev., 34: 619–642.

Clark, E. R., and E. L. Clark 1935 Observations on changes in blood vascular endothelium in the living animal. Am. J. Anat., 57: 384–438.

Cunningham, R. S. 1924 Physiology of endothelial cells. Am. Rev. Tuberculosis, 9: 941.

Danielli, J. F., and A. Stock 1944 Structure and permeability of blood capillaries. Biol. Rev., 19: 81–94.

Franklin, K. J. 1937 A Monograph on Veins. Charles Thomas, Springfield, Illinois.

166

Hughes, A. F. N.   1935   The elongation of previously rounded endothelial cell nuclei as an
index of the tensions which are present in the
cell. J. Anat., 70: 76. 122.

Mehrotra, R. M. L.   1953   An experimental
study of the changes which occur in ligated
arteries and veins. J. Path. Bact., 65: 2.

O'Neill, J. F.   1947   The effects on venous endothelium of alterations in blood flow through the
vessels in vein walls, and the possible relation
to thrombosis. Ann. Surg., 126: 270–288.

Samuels, P. B., B. M. Samuels and D. R. Webster
1952   New techniques in the study of venous
endothelium. J. Lab. Invest., 1: 1.

PLATE 1

EXPLANATION OF FIGURES

1 Endothelial nuclei of tibialis vein of the grassfrog (*Rana pipiens*). Harris' hematoxylin and eosin. × 900.

2 Same as figure 1. × 400.

3 Endothelial nuclei of tibialis vein of the bullfrog (*Rana catesbiana*). Harris' hemotoxylin and eosin. × 900.

4 Endothelial nuclei of the lower femoral vein of the dog. Harris' hematoxylin and eosin. × 900.

5 Endothelial nuclei of the lower femoral vein of the guinea pig. Harris' hematoxylin and eosin. × 900.

6 Endothelial nuclei of the tibialis vein of the rabbit. Harris' hematoxylin and eosin. × 900.

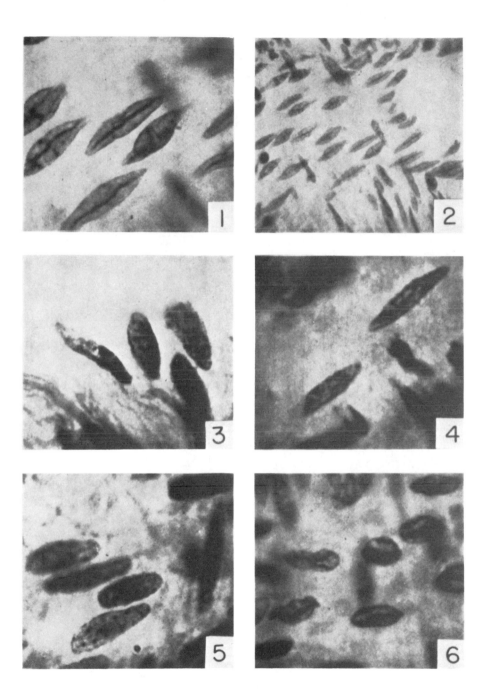

PLATE 2

7 Cross section of relaxed femoral vein of dog. Harris' hematoxylin and eosin. $\times$ 420.

8 Cross section of constricted guinea pig tibialis vein. Harris' hematoxylin and eosin. $\times$ 900.

9 Cross section of femoral vein of bullfrog. Harris' hematoxylin and eosin. $\times$ 400.

10 Cross section of constricted tibialis vein of pigeon. Harris' hematoxylin and eosin. $\times$ 800.

11 Cross section of lateral branch of constricted saphenous vein in the cow. Verhoeff and Van Gieson. $\times$ 200.

12 Cross section of partially constricted metatarsal vein of cow. Harris' hematoxylin and eosin. $\times$ 400.

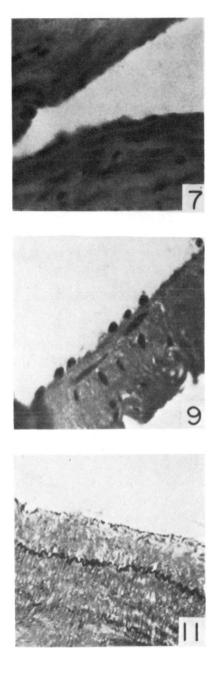
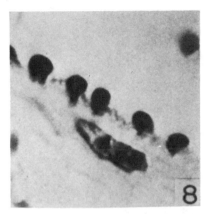
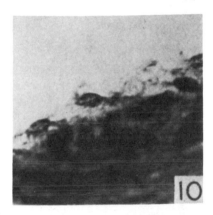
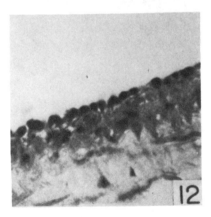

Ultrastructure

THE FINE STRUCTURE OF YOUNG AND OLD SPINAL GANGLIA [1]

ARTHUR HESS [2]

SEVENTEEN FIGURES

Despite the intensive studies devoted to the structure of nerve cell bodies and the extracellular and intracellular elements associated with them, there are still many aspects of the structural organization of the cells of the spinal ganglia awaiting final resolution.

It has been suggested that there are various nerve cell types in spinal ganglia, and some authors have even assigned different functional properties to these cells based on a histological study of sections with the light microscope (see Bacsich and Wyburn, '53). The disposition of the Nissl bodies, mitochondria, and Golgi apparatus in these cells has occupied much attention (Beams, van Breemen, Newfang and Evans, '52). The satellite cells of the ganglion also have been investigated. In addition, the ageing of nerve cells and the accumulation of lipofuchsin pigment (Andrew, '52) has been observed frequently.

In this study of spinal ganglia, we have attempted, through the application of ultrathin sectioning and electron microscopy to:

(1) ascertain the possible occurrence of cell types and characterize morphologically the basis for any such cell variants;

[1] This investigation was supported in part by research grants B-341 and B-425 from the Institute of Neurological Diseases and Blindness of the National Institutes of Health, Public Health Service.

[2] With the technical assistance of Charles E. Houck, Jr. and Emil C. Sanders.

(2) study the fine structure of the karyoplasm, nucleolus, and cytoplasm or neuroplasm;

(3) resolve further the structure of Nissl bodies or chromophil substance;

(4) determine the disposition and structure of mitochondria;

(5) study the occurrence and structure of the Golgi apparatus;

(6) study the morphology of the satellite cells and their relationship to the spinal ganglion nerve cells and to each other;

(7) investigate in senile animals the spinal ganglion cells, their mitochondria and the distribution and fine structure of the pigment and to draw some conclusions as to the probable mechanism of its formation.

MATERIAL AND METHODS

The spinal ganglia of guinea pigs were used. The animals were divided roughly into three groups: (1) *young* animals of three days of age; (2) *adult* animals that had given birth to at least one litter; (3) *old* or *senile* animals of 6 years of age. These latter animals were donated generously by Dr. James B. Rogers of the Department of Anatomy, University of Louisville School of Medicine, Louisville, Kentucky, to whom we are very grateful.

The techniques were essentially the same as those used previously for the study of the fine structure of peripheral nerve fibers (Hess and Lansing, '53). The spinal ganglia, dissected most frequently from thoracic vertebral levels, were placed in Dalton's fixative (Dalton and Felix, '55) for one-half to two hours. Most of the sections examined were obtained from material allowed to fix for one and one-half hours. The ganglia then were washed in distilled water and placed in 70% alcohol, dehydrated and embedded in a mixture of partially polymerized butyl and methyl methacrylate. A few ganglia were also fixed in buffered osmic acid (Palade, '52a), varying in concentration from 1% to 3% and containing mammalian Ringer's solution, for 4 hours, then similarly treated as above. The fixation yielded by Dalton's fluid was vastly superior. Previous studies in this laboratory have shown that nerve tissue has a predilection to swell and "explode" during the embedding process. The use of partially polymerized plastic for embedding usually prevents this, although it does not invariably yield perfect results.

Sections were made and mounted on copper mesh grids, which were then inserted into an RCA-EMU type microscope. Negatives were exposed at a magnification of 1000 to 6000 × and photographically enlarged.

To facilitate identification of the cellular elements and to determine the location in the ganglia of the section under observation in the electron microscope, thin plastic sections were studied in the phase-contrast microscope. Reference was also made to cytological and neurohistological frozen and paraffin preparations of spinal ganglia to correlate observations made with the light and electron microscopes.

RESULTS

Spinal ganglion nerve cells

Cell types. In ganglia from guinea pigs of all ages, two distinct cell types are found (fig. 1). In one, the cells are small, the cytoplasm is very osmophilic, and the ground substance or neuroplasm of the cell is well organized; the chromophil substance extends evenly throughout the cell (fig. 15). In the other cell type, the cells are large, the intensity of osmophilia is low, the Nissl substance is easily recognized and organized into scattered clumps or bodies (fig. 7). That this is a real difference and is not necessarily a factor induced by fixation can be seen by observing these two cell variants in juxtaposition to one another. The main difference between these two cell types resides in the distribution of the Nissl substance, with the first or "dark" type of cell having chromophil substance extending throughout the length and breadth of the cell, thus giving high electron density to

177

the cytoplasm; while the second or "light" type of cell has Nissl substance distributed in discrete clumps and producing in general a low electron density of the cytoplasm.

There are transitional cell types with density of cytoplasm and of cytoplasmic elements ranging in intensity between the "dark" and "light" cell variants (fig. 1). However, the "dark" and "light" cell types as indicated above are representative of such a dichotomy in spinal ganglion nerve cells.

The remaining items will be discussed in relation to the cell types, and the differences, if any, in the morphology or disposition of the elements under consideration will be noted.

Nucleus and nucleolus. The nucleoplasm of spinal ganglion cells is sparse and irregularly dispersed (fig. 16). The nucleus possesses a typical double membrane (figs. 15 and 16). The nucleolus is very dense and consists of at least three components (fig. 16). One is a vesicular component with filaments enclosing small vacuoles and is the most prominent part of the nucleolus. Another portion of the nucleolus, most frequently intimately associated with the filamentous structure, is a dense irregular mass yielding mainly a homogeneous appearance with only a few large granules. Other irregular masses, presenting a more granular appearance than the former and less dense, comprise the third component of the nucleolus.

Any one of these three nucleolar components can be found adherent or closer to the nuclear membrane than the others (fig. 9), yielding an appearance similar to that of the nucleolar satellite (Barr, Bertram and Lindsay, '50); we have no information as to its significance.

There are no differences in the cell types of nucleus or nucleolus. The nucleolar satellite body also appears in both cell types.

Cell membrane. The limiting cell membrane of the spinal ganglion nerve cell presents a structure similar to the membranes of other cells. It is rather difficult to define its exact structure and dimensions since the satellite cell, to be discussed later, is in juxtaposition with it.

178

Most frequently, the nerve cell membrane is smooth. However, often it reveals thin villiform projections extending outward from the nerve cell surface (fig. 7). The margins of these processes are continuous with the cell membrane. The less dense central portion of these projections has the same density as the nerve cell cytoplasm, so that these villiform projections are true processes of the nerve cell. The projections are also seen cut in cross-section. They are probably due to the harsh treatment accorded the nerve cell by fixation.

Neurofibrils. We have seen no structure in the cytoplasm that can be interpreted as a neurofibril. Indeed, the opposite view is probably true in that there appears to be no orientation in the cytoplasm, either of the neuroplasm itself or of the distribution of the cytoplasmic elements, except for the internal organization of the Nissl substance discussed below. The fibrillar structures mentioned by Beams et al. ('52) as neurofibrils do not appear in our material.

Chromophil substance. The observation that Nissl bodies contain ribonucleoprotein suggests that this substance should appear morphologically similar to the structural system described as "endoplasmic reticulum" by Palade and Porter ('54), "ergastoplasm" by Weiss ('53), and double-membraned system by Weiss and Lansing ('53). Although none of these terms is entirely appropriate for nerve tissue, the term "ergastoplasm" will be used in this paper. The latter presumably corresponnds to the basophilic material in cytoplasm (Bernhard, Haguenau, Gautier and Oberling, '52). Haguenau and Bernhard ('53) have described Nissl material in nerve cells with the use of the electron microscope.

When the Nissl substance is viewed under relatively low magnification, it appears as a densely-packed mass of small granules (figs. 7 and 15). However, with higher magnification, some of the granules can be resolved as very fine tubular filaments surrounded by granules (figs. 11 and 14). This is an appearance similar to endoplasmic reticulum or ergastoplasm previously described in nerve tissue (Hess and

Lansing, '53). The tubular filaments are in layers, one placed on top of the other. The granules are perhaps more numerous than those of ergastoplasm in other cells. At higher magnifications, the granules are seen to have smaller, denser granules in and around them, yielding a punctate appearance. In addition, the granules associated with the tubular filaments are usually not only aligned against the filaments, but also frequently can be found evenly-spaced in a row between the filaments. The tubular elements of each Nissl body are also highly oriented, so that in a mass of Nissl, all the components are sectioned in the same direction. One Nissl body may have its tubules cut neatly in cross-section; while in an adjacent clump of Nissl, all the units may be cut tangentially.

Clumps of Nissl substance appear only in "light" cells; aggregations occur throughout the cytoplasm of "dark" cells. However, even though the distribution of chromophil substance differs in the two cell types, the units composing the Nissl substance are the same (figs. 11 and 14).

Mitochondria. The mitochondria are small, thin, and elongated and possess the cristae or folds characteristic of this organelle (figs. 7, 11 and 15). They are, in principle, similar to mitochondria previously described (Palade, '52b; Hess and Lansing, '53). Higher magnifications reveal at times that the folds of mitochondria do not pass across the entire width of the mitochondrion, but are seen cut in cross-section (fig. 12). The haphazard arrangement of the folds in the interior of the mitochondrion indicate that perhaps the main folds possess villous extensions. Y-shaped and T-shaped bifurcating mitochondria have also been noticed.

One is impressed by the relatively small diameter of several of the mitochondria in these nerve cells. As an approximation, several of them are as little as one-half the diameter of the mitochondria in many tissue cells. Another point worthy of note is the close packing and large number of mitochondrial folds. While this is by no means diagnostic for

Nucleus. The nucleoplasm of the satellite cell usually presents a more or less homogeneous appearance with the dense chromatin material dispersed throughout the nucleus (fig. 17). At times, the chromatin material is not so evenly dispersed and is aggregated into several irregular clumps (fig. 8). The nucleoplasm is much more dense than that of the nerve cell.

The satellite cell nucleus is usually intimately related to the nerve cell. It is either separated from the nerve cell by its own intervening cytoplasm or rests on the nerve cell, giving the appearance of a demilune. Frequently, the satellite cell nucleus has a more intimate relation to the nerve cell and causes an indentation in the cytoplasm of the nerve cell (fig. 5).

Cytoplasm. The cytoplasm of the satellite cell is very difficult to fix. It frequently tears away from the nerve cell. At times, it appears relatively devoid of formed elements. However, favorable preparations reveal that the cytoplasm is fairly dense, containing scattered ergastoplasmic filaments and granules and mitochondria that compare in size with those of the nerve cell (fig. 8).

The satellite cell cytoplasm completely surrounds the nerve cell, even though at times it appears thin and attenuated (figs. 11 and 15).

Cell membrane. The limiting membrane of the satellite cell presents the structure typical of other cells (figs. 8, 11, and 15). The cell membrane of these cells can be divided into two parts — that apposed to the ganglion nerve cell and the surface distal to the nerve cell. Both surfaces are usually relatively smooth, the former following the contour of the ganglion cell and the latter, the surface of satellite cells belonging to neighboring nerve cells or the outlines of an intervening connective tissue capsule (figs. 11 and 15).

However, a frequent occurrence, usually near the nucleus of the satellite cell, is the appearance of a collection of membranes (figs. 13 and 17). These membranes, each of about the same thickness as the limiting membrane of the satellite cell elsewhere, twist and fold, establishing a complex labyrinthine apparatus. There are at least two relationships of satellite cells that could account for this appearance. One is that the varied membrane appearance is due to extensive overlapping of processes of satellite cells belonging to one nerve cell and serving to form its capsule. The other view is that the complex apparatus represents local meanderings of the membranes themselves of one satellite cell. Although not definitely established, we at present tend to favor the latter viewpoint. Evidence for this is that it is possible in some sections to trace some of the membranous folds back to the surface membrane of the satellite cell. It can then be seen that both surfaces of the satellite cell membrane, that apposed to the nerve cell and that distal from it, contribute to the complex membranous apparatus. Another point in favor of this view is that the complex membranous apparatus occurs frequently near the nucleus of a satellite cell. Since the nucleus of the satellite cell is located centrally in the light microscope with approximately equal amounts of cytoplasm extending from it, the location of the complex membranous apparatus near the nucleus would indicate that it is formed locally by the membranes of one cell. Of course, it is not impossible that the overlap of cytoplasm of the satellite cells belonging to a single neuron is so extensive that processes of satellite cells can extend for long distances and reach as far as the centrally-located nucleus of an adjacent satellite cell belonging to the same neuron, yielding the folded membrane appearance.

The various relationships and appearances of the satellite cell do not appear to be restricted to a single nerve cell type, but can usually be found in relation to "dark" or "light" cells.

There are similarities between satellite cells, Schwann cells, and neuroglia. The similarities in the relationships of perineuronal glial satellites and nerve cells of the central nervous system (see Penfield, '32) and the satellite cells and spinal ganglion nerve cells described here are striking. The nucleus and the cytoplasmic contents of the satellite cells are similar to those of Schwann cells (Hess and Lansing, '53). The indentation of the cytoplasm of the spinal ganglion cell caused by the satellite cell nucleus is reminiscent of the indenting of the axon and myelin sheath by the Schwann cell nucleus (Hess and Lansing, '53). Since the neurilemma includes the membrane of the Schwann cell (Hess, '55) and is a continuous sheath throughout the extent of the peripheral nerve fiber, the Schwann cell of adjacent internodal segments can be considered as forming a syncitium across the node of Ranvier, even though the Schwann cell cytoplasm might appear arrested at the node. Satellite cell cytoplasm surrounds the spinal ganglion nerve cell. Among histologists, the prevailing view is that the satellite cells are continuous with the neurilemma at the region of exit of the nerve process and that the satellite and Schwann cells have a common origin from the neural crest (see Singer, '54). Thus the spinal ganglion cell and its process that enters the peripheral nerve (its dendrite) are enclosed in a continuous sheath of cells. Rio-Hortega also believed in the similarities of neuroglia, satellite cells, and Schwann cells and called the latter two "peripheral neuroglia" (see Penfield, '32).

Senile spinal ganglion nerve cells

Degeneration of cells, of course, may be found in senile ganglia and these will manifest hyperchromatic nuclei, chromatolysis, etc. (see Andrew, '52). In cells that are not in the process of degeneration, the cell membrane, nuclear membrane, nucleoli, and Nissl substance do not exhibit obvious age changes. The accumulation of pigment, however, is a characteristic of all senile spinal ganglion nerve cells. In addition, it is also necessary to comment on the structure of the mitochondria since these organelles have been described as undergoing profound alterations in structure with age (Payne, '52; Weiss and Lansing, '53).

Mitochondria. Characteristic mitochondria, as found in nerve tissue (Hess and Lansing, '53), are found in spinal ganglion nerve cells with and without obvious age changes. Thus, apparently intact mitochondria are found in ganglion cells containing dense accumulations of pigment (fig. 4). The mitochondria, exhibiting normal folds, are scattered at random throughout the cytoplasm. However, we have also observed swollen and vacuolated mitochondria in senile spinal ganglion cells (fig. 3). These mitochondria conform closely to the description of Weiss and Lansing ('53) in their paper on the age changes of the anterior pituitary of the mouse. The mitochondria are several times enlarged and rounded; the matrix material is essentially lacking or very dilute as evidenced by lack of density within the mitochondria. The folds are barely recognizable as very short inward extensions from the limiting membrane or surface of the mitochondria. It is interesting to note that both the apparently intact mitochondria and the degenerative mitochondria are found in cells that appear well-fixed. This gives rise to the implication that at least some ganglion cells exhibit mitochondrial ageing (Payne, '52; Weiss and Lansing, '53). However, we have found comparable degenerative mitochondria in sections of very young (three-day-old) and adult spinal ganglion cells of guinea pigs in which pigment was absent and no age changes had occurred (fig. 13). Since degenerative mitochondria can be found in young and adult cells and normal mitochondria are seen in senile cells, it is difficult, at least for individual spinal ganglion cells, to use the condition of the mitochondria as an index of ageing.

Pigment. In the extremely senile guinea pigs we have studied, virtually all of the ganglion cells, despite cell type, contain pigment bodies in varying amounts (figs. 4 and 6). The pigment usually tends to form aggregations toward the periphery and more frequently occurs around the entire border of the cell, rather than in its interior.

The pigment bodies are characterized by very marked electron density and vary in shape from spheroidal to highly irregular bodies. Their density approximates that of lipoidal inclusions or nucleolar material. Although the most frequent appearance is that of a homogeneous mass, there are not uncommon exceptions. The pigment bodies are usually dense and solid (figs. 4 and 10). However, in some instances, the pigment body seems to be composed of a number of vesicles of very low electron density surrounded by a lacework of dense material (fig. 6). In still other instances, the combination of the aforementioned forms occurs with the pigment body being composed of both solid and vesiculated forms (fig. 6). Vesicles can vary from one to many in a pigment body.

Beginning pigment formation seems to occur in most intimate relation with swollen mitochondria (figs. 2 and 10). This relation of mitochondria and pigment is seen not only in senile cells (fig. 2), but also in adult animals (fig. 10) where only infrequent cells exhibit small amounts of pigment. The mitochondria swell, their borders become very dense, and the internal folds disappear with the interior of the mitochondria assuming a homogeneous, less dense appearance. The pigment granules accumulate in relation to the mitochondria and extend from one pole of the mitochondria. Payne ('52) has observed that one of the first changes in ageing mitochondria is that "they appear as brown pigment-like bodies." The accumulation of pigment apparently progresses by the formation of a successive series of vesicles which then coalesce to form a pigment body. A suggested series of stages in the formation of a pigment body is presented in figures 2, 6 and 4.

SUMMARY

Ultrathin sections were made of the spinal ganglia of three-day-old, adult, and 6-year-old guinea pigs and examined with the electron microscope. Two nerve cell types are observed, mainly based on the distribution of the Nissl substance. The nucleoplasm and three components of the nucleolus of the neurons are described. The cell membrane of the nerve cell can be smooth or can present thin villiform projections

185

containing nerve cytoplasm. No evidence of neurofibrils is seen. Nissl substance is composed of layers of fine tubular filaments with granules apposed to them and lined up between them, similar to the appearance of ergastoplasm in other cells. The tubular elements of a Nissl body are oriented in one direction. The mitochondria are usually small, thin, and elongated and present numerous, closely-spaced folds. The main folds might present villous extensions. A structure similar to the Golgi apparatus of other cells occurs extensively throughout the cell and can be found near the nucleus and near the limiting cell membrane. It consists of membranes, granules, and vacuoles and is similar to that described in other cells.

The nucleus of the satellite cell is described. It can cause an indentation in the nerve cell cytoplasm. The satellite cell cytoplasm contains mitochondria and scattered ergastoplasmic filaments and granules. It encapsulates the neurons. The membrane of the satellite cell is described. A complex membranous apparatus, produced either by invagination and folding of the membrane of a single satellite cell or by overlapping of the processes of adjacent satellite cells, has been found, usually located near the satellite cell nucleus. A discussion is presented concerning the significance of and comparing morphological similarities of satellite cells, Schwann cells, and neuroglia.

Degenerative mitochondria can be found in young and adult nerve cells and normal mitochondria are seen in senile cells. It is difficult to use the condition of the mitochondria as an index of ageing. All senile ganglion nerve cells present pigment. The appearance and distribution of the pigment bodies are described. A suggested series of stages of pigment formation, arising from swollen mitochondria, is presented.

LITERATURE CITED

ANDREW, W. 1952 Cellular Changes With Age. Springfield, Illinois; Charles C Thomas. 74 pp.

BACSICH, P., AND G. M. WYBURN 1953 Formalin-sensitive cells in spinal ganglia. Quart. Journ. Micr. Sci., *94:* 89–92.

BARR, M. L., L. F. BERTRAM AND H. A. LINDSAY 1950 The morphology of the nerve cell nucleus, according to sex. Anat. Rec., *107*: 283–298.

BEAMS, H. W., V. L. VAN BREEMEN, D. M. NEWFANG AND T. C. EVANS 1952 A correlated study on spinal ganglion cells and associated nerve fibers with the light and electron microscopes. J. Comp. Neur., *96*: 249–281.

BERNHARD, W., F. HAGUENAU, A. GAUTIER AND C. OBERLIN 1952 La structure submicroscopique des elements basophiles cytoplasmiques dans le foie, le pancreas et les glandes salivaires. Z. Zellforschg. mikr. Anat., *37*: 281–300.

DALTON, A. J., AND M. D. FELIX 1955 A study of the Golgi substance and ergastoplasm in a series of mammalian cell types. Exp. Cell Res. In press.

HAGUENAU, F., AND W. BERNHARD 1953 Aspect de la substance de Nissl au microscope électronique. Exp. Cell Res., *4*: 496–498.

HESS, A. 1955 The fine structure and morphological organization of non-myelinated nerve fibres. Proc. Roy. Soc. B. (in press).

HESS, A., AND A. I. LANSING 1953 The fine structure of peripheral nerve fibers. Anat. Rec., *117*: 175–200.

PALADE, G. E. 1952a A study of fixation for electron microscopy. J. Exp. Med., *95*: 285–298.

————— 1952b The fine structure of mitochondria. Anat. Rec., *114*: 427–451.

PALADE, G. E., AND K. R. PORTER 1954 Studies on the endoplasmic reticulum. I. Its indentification in cells *in situ*. J. Exp. Med., *100*: 641–656.

PAYNE, F. 1952 Cytological changes in the cells of the pituitary, thyroids, adrenals and sex glands of ageing fowl, p. 381–402. In Cowdry's Problems of Ageing, Third Edition, edited by A. I. Lansing. Williams and Wilkins Co.: Baltimore.

PENFIELD, W. 1932 Neuroglia. Normal and Pathological. In Cytology and Cellular Pathology of the Nervous System, vol. II, p. 421–479. New York: Paul B. Hoeber, Inc.

SINGER, M. 1954 Nervous system, p. 194–272. In Histology, edited by R. O. Greep. New York: Blakiston Co., Inc.

SJÖSTRAND, F. S., AND V. HANZON 1954 Ultrastructure of Golgi apparatus of exocrine cells of mouse pancreas. Exp. Cell Res., *7*: 415–429.

WEISS, J. M. 1953 The ergastoplasm. J. Exp. Med., *98*: 607–618.

WEISS, J., AND A. I. LANSING 1953 Age changes in the fine structure of anterior pituitary of the mouse. Proc. Soc. Exp. Biol. and Med., *82*: 460–466.

All illustrations are electron micrographs of the spinal ganglia of guinea pigs. All magnifications are approximate. The photographs of this plate are from ganglia fixed in Palade's ('52a) fluid.

1   Spinal ganglion nerve cells illustrating the nerve cell types with varying densities of cytoplasm. × 1000.

2   Apparently swollen mitochondrion (M) in intimate relation with the supposed beginning of pigment (P) formation. × 12000.

3   A neuron of a senile guinea pig showing swollen degenerative mitochondria (M) and pigment (P). × 12,000.

4   A neuron of a senile guinea pig illustrating solid and dense pigment bodies (P) and intact mitochondria (M). × 12,000.

5.   A nerve cell and satellite cell nucleus showing the latter causing an indentation in the neuron cytoplasm. × 3000.

6   Neuron cytoplasm of a senile guinea pig showing vesiculated bodies (P) believed to be various stages in the formation of the pigment. × 12000.

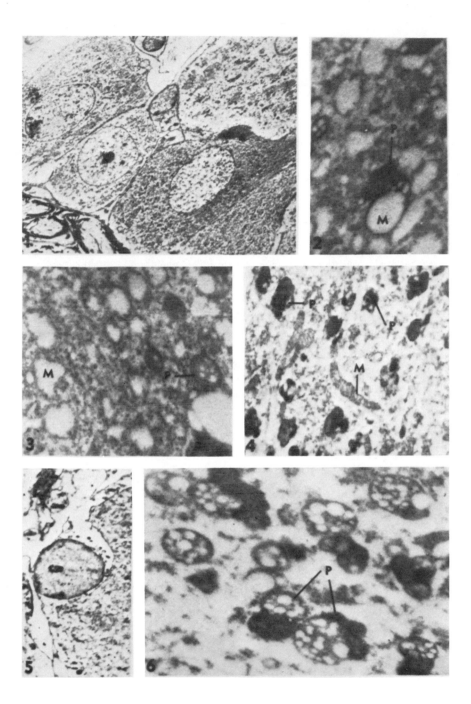

PLATE 2

EXPLANATION OF FIGURES

All illustrations are electron micrographs of the spinal ganglia of guinea pigs. All magnifications are approximate. The photographs of this plate are from ganglia fixed in Dalton's (Dalton and Felix, '55) fluid.

7 A "light" ganglion cell with clumped Nissl substance and villiform processes extending from the cell membrane. The Golgi apparatus (G) is seen near the cell membrane. A mitochondrion (M) is also shown. × 15000.

8 A satellite cell nucleus with clumped chromatin. The satellite cell cytoplasm contains mitochondria and scattered ergastoplasmic filaments and granules. The satellite cell limiting membrane can also be seen. × 15000.

9 Part of the nucleolus near the nuclear membrane of the nerve cell yielding the appearance of a nucleolar satellite. × 15000.

10 An adult nerve cell showing beginning pigment (P) formation extending from the pole of swollen mitochondria (M). × 15000.

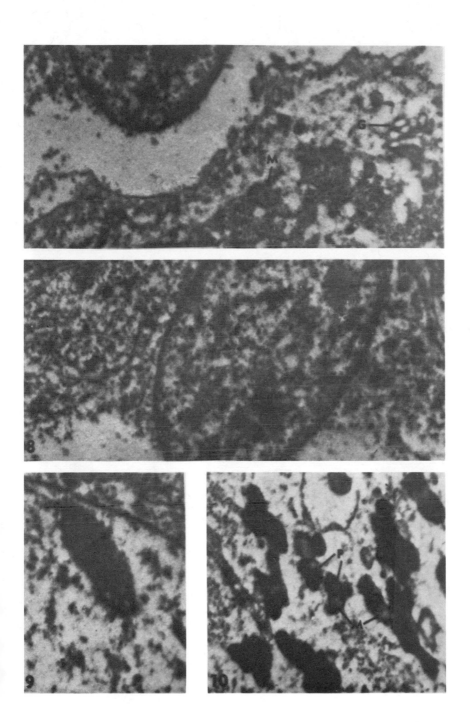

All illustrations are electron micrographs of the spinal ganglia of guinea pigs. All magnifications are approximate. The photographs of this plate are from ganglia fixed in Dalton's (Dalton and Felix, '55) fluid.

11 An illustration of the cytoplasmic contents of the "dark" cell type showing the similarity of the Nissl substance to ergastoplasm (E), ergastoplasmic filaments and punctate granules apposed to and lined in a row between the filaments, the Golgi apparatus (G) near the limiting membrane and mitochondria (M). The thin satellite cell cytoplasm (SC) encapsulates the neuron. The satellite cell limiting membrane is also shown. × 24000.

12 An enlargement of figure 11 showing the Golgi apparatus with Golgi vacuoles (Gv), membranes (Gm), and granules (Gg). The villous folds of a mitochondrion (M) are also shown. × 42000.

192

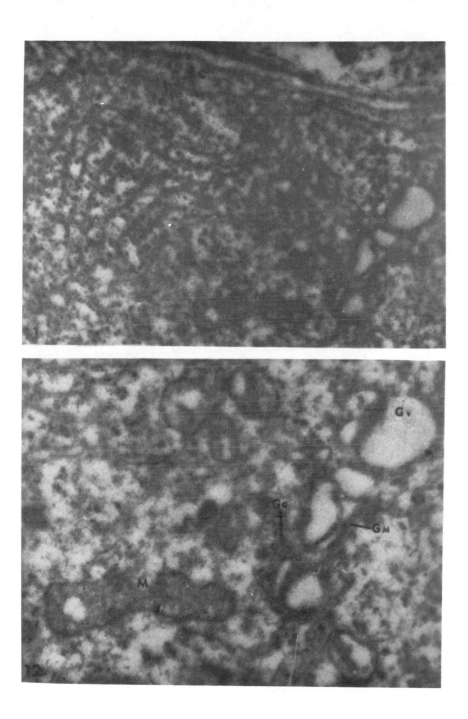

193

PLATE 4

EXPLANATION OF FIGURES

All illustrations are electron micrographs of the spinal ganglia of guinea pigs. All magnifications are approximate. The photographs of this plate are from ganglia fixed in Dalton's (Dalton and Felix, '55) fluid.

13 The complex membranous apparatus (MA) of the satellite cell cytoplasm is shown. The adult nerve cell has some swollen degenerative mitochondria (M). × 15000.

14 A Nissl body of a "light" cell is shown and is similar to ergastoplasm with layers of filaments and granules between them. × 20000.

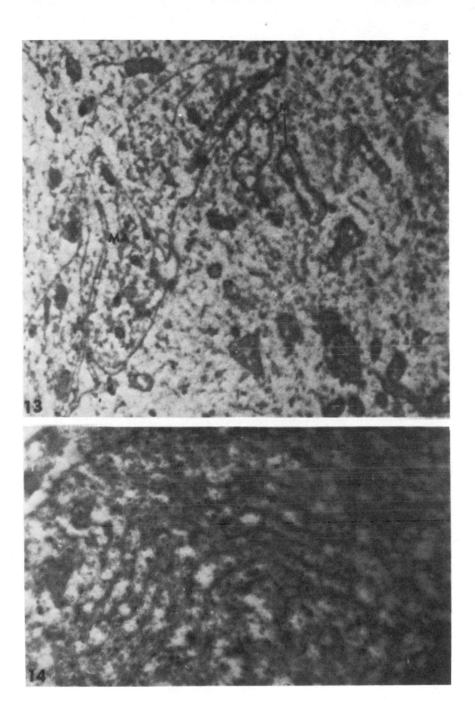

PLATE 5

All illustrations are electron micrographs of the spinal ganglia of guinea pigs. All magnifications are approximate. The photographs of this plate are from ganglia fixed in Dalton's (Dalton and Felix, '55) fluid.

15 Cytoplasm of a "dark" cell showing the diffuse and scattered Nissl substance, Golgi apparatus (G) near the nerve cell nucleus (MN), and mitochondria (M). The double-walled structure of the nerve cell nuclear membrane is shown. The satellite cell cytoplasm (SC) encapsulates the neuron. The satellite cell limiting membrane can also be seen. × 20000.

16 A nerve cell nucleus showing the vesicular part of the nucleolus (N_1), the irregular homogenous mass commonly associated with it (N_2), and the other irregular punctate masses (N_3). The membrane of the nerve cell nucleus is also shown. × 12000.

17 The complex membranous apparatus (MA) of the satellite cell cytoplasm is shown near the satellite cell nucleus (SN). The satellite cell nucleus is more or less homogeneous in appearance. × 15000.

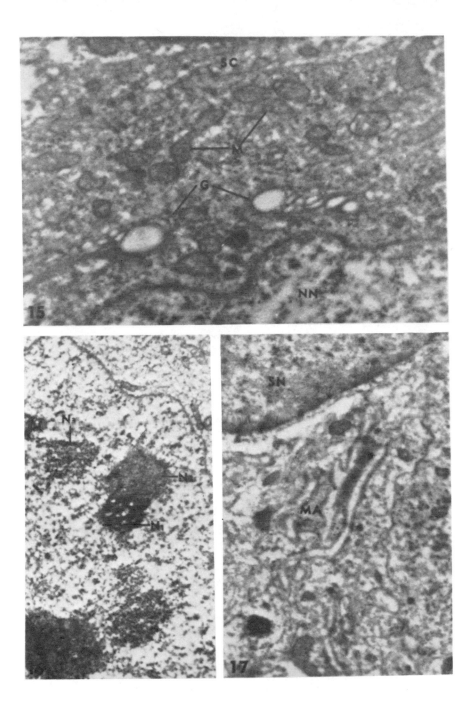

Neurosecretion-like Material in the Hindbrain of Ageing Sheep and Sheep affected with Natural Scrapie

A. Bignami
Elisabeth Beck
H. B. Parry

The earliest lesion in the cerebellum of sheep affected with natural scrapie is a degeneration of the mossy terminals within the granular layer of the cerebellar cortex[1,2]. With this in mind we have made a combined electron and light microscope study of these early lesions. We used sheep from a supervised breeding population, the normal controls being genetically non-susceptible to natural scrapie[3].

A 4 yr old female sheep, affected with natural scrapie, .was perfused with 4 per cent glutaraldehyde in a phosphate buffer adjusted to pH 7·3. Thin slices were then removed from various parts of the cerebellum and from the supraoptic nucleus of the hypothalamus. The specimens were post-fixed in phosphate buffered osmium tetroxide, dehydrated, stained in 1 per cent uranyl acetate and embedded in 'Epon' in flat-foil dishes. Grids containing ribbons of sections were stained with lead citrate and examined with an AEI electron microscope. The rest of the brain was post-fixed in 10 per cent formol-saline. Light microscopy of the cerebellum revealed a moderate number of degenerated mossy terminals within the granule layer of the nodule (Fig. 1A) and some swellings (torpedoes) on the axons of Purkinje cells in other parts of the vermis. Apart from these changes, there was a slight fibrillary gliosis, confined to the nodule, but no obvious reduction in the number of Purkinje or granule cells.

Electron microscopy of the cerebellum revealed that the pathological lesions were essentially confined to the granule layer of the nodule. Here accumulations of dense bodies, varying in shape and size, and of dense core vesicles 40–100 nm in diameter, were seen within both mossy terminals and fine unmyelinated nerve processes (Fig. 2A). The appearance of such accumulations within fine unmyelinated nerve processes was reminiscent of electron micrographs of Herring corpuscles in the pituitary stalk of normal dogs[4]; here these accumulations are interpreted as neurosecretory material. (Similar accumulations of dense bodies were also found within fine nerve processes

of the degenerated supraoptic nucleus of the hypothalamo-neurohypophysial system in the present case;
Fig. 2B.)

In view of the morphological similarities between the
electron microscopical appearance of fine unmyelinated
fibres in the cerebellum and the hypothalamus of our case,
sections of cerebellum embedded in paraffin were treated
so as to show up the neurosecretory material (Bargmann's
modification of Gomori's chrome–alum–haematoxylin
(CAH) and performic acid–alcian blue (PFAB)). These
sections had small deposits of CAH and PFAB positive
material (Fig. 1B) in regions which also had degenerated
mossy terminals. Further tests to determine the properties
of this "neurosecretory" material showed that the PFAB
reaction was abolished when oxidation was omitted. It
remained grossly unchanged after lipid extraction,
however. The material also remained unaffected by digestion with trypsin. The latter test alone distinguishes it
from neurosecretory material as found in the hypothalamo-
neurohypophysial system where the reaction is negative
after incubation in trypsin[5,6]. Reactions for lipofuscin
and neutral fat were negative.

Deposits of CAH and PFAB positive material and, in
sections impregnated with silver, degenerated *boutons
terminaux*, were also found in other parts of the hindbrain,
that is, the pontine nuclei (Fig. 3A), inferior olives, lateral
cuneate and lateral reticular nuclei—all regions with
cerebellar connexions which frequently degenerate in
natural scrapie[1].

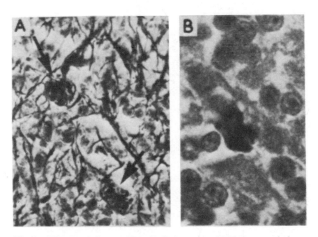

Fig. 1. Degenerated mossy terminals (arrows) within the granule layer
of the cerebellum in (A) a sheep affected with natural scrapie (Marsland-
Glees silver impregnation, × 480), and (B) CAH positive deposit in the
same location in another animal with scrapie (Gomori chrome–alum–
haematoxylin stain, × 1,200); note the shape of the CAH positive
deposit which closely resembles that of the degenerated mossy terminal.

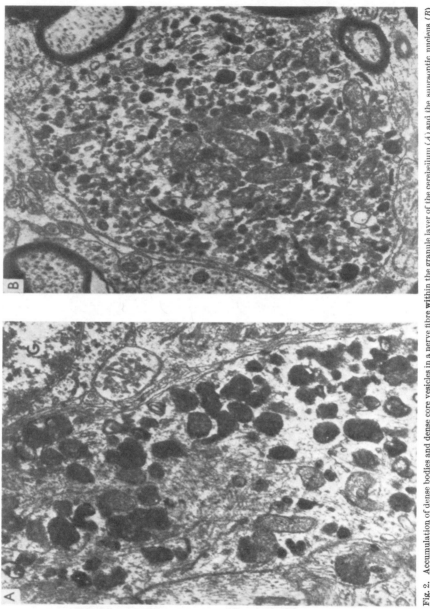

Fig. 2.   Accumulation of dense bodies and dense core vesicles in a nerve fibre within the granule layer of the cerebellum (A) and the supraoptic nucleus (B) of a sheep affected with scrapie.   Note the similarity in the morphological appearance.   G, Granule cell.   (× 24,000.)

The cerebellum and brain stem nuclei of fourteen more sheep affected with natural scrapie ($2\frac{1}{2}$–$4\frac{1}{2}$ yr old), and seven normal controls of both sexes (10 months to 10 yr old), were examined under the light microscope for the presence of "neurosecretory" material. In the scrapie group numerous deposits of CAH and PFAB positive material were found, in both the granule layer of the cerebellum and the brain stem nuclei with cerebellar connexions, when degenerated nerve fibres and terminals were prominent; that is, in the early stages of degeneration. In animals with more advanced degeneration, showing a loss of nerve cells and dense fibrous gliosis[1], such material was either absent or present in small quantities. The younger controls tended to have no or very little CAH and PFAB positive material, while an increasing amount, sometimes comparable with that observed in the early stages of scrapie, was found in older animals (Fig. 3B).

To determine the precise location of the "neurosecretory" material, sections well supplied with it were first impregnated with silver, then photographed, bleached and stained with CAH. In this way it was often possible to demonstrate CAH positive material at the site of a degenerating mossy ending or bouton terminal.

Because "neurosecretory" material was more abundant in old sheep, one normal, old female sheep ($7\frac{1}{4}$ yr old) was perfused with glutaraldehyde for electron microscopy. Dense bodies and dense core vesicles were found within the terminals and fine nerve fibres of the pontine nuclei and the inferior olives. Light microscopy revealed CAH and PFAB positive deposits in the same nuclei. Such deposits were rare in the cerebellum and no attempt was made to see them with the electron microscope.

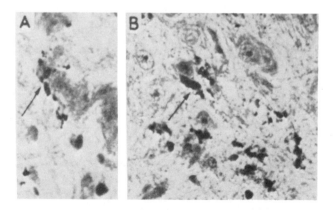

Fig. 3. CAH positive substance shown as dark, irregular deposits (arrows) in the pontine nuclei of a sheep affected with scrapie (*A*) and in those of a normal sheep 7·5 yr old (*B*). Note in *A* the close apposition of the deposits to a nerve cell, simulating degenerated *boutons terminaux*. (Gomori chrome–alum–haematoxylin stain. *A*, × 770; *B*, × 480.)

It is now well established that the material stained by CAH and PFAB in the hypothalamo-neurohypophysial system is rich in protein-bound cystine or cysteine[5]; it is regarded by some[7] as a bearer substance for the hormones of the posterior pituitary gland, although this is a controversial interpretation[8]. The presence of a similarly staining material in the hindbrain of ageing sheep and sheep affected with scrapie therefore does not imply that hormones of the posterior lobe are to be found in this location, or that this material is true neurosecretion in the sense that it is released into the blood stream. But our findings suggest that substances similar to those produced by the neurones of the supraoptic and paraventricular nuclei of the hypothalamus, and with similar tinctorial properties, may also be elaborated by certain other groups of nerve cells throughout the nervous system. We noted that, except for the oldest controls when the distribution was rather more diffuse, the greatest concentrations of CAH and PFAB positive material were confined to brain stem nuclei with cerebellar connexions and to the cerebellar cortex itself. (The distribution in other regions of the brain is now being examined.)

We cannot determine yet whether this CAH and PFAB positive material is a normal product of the nerve cell which, because of "irreversible disturbance of flow"[8] or increased synthesis, accumulates at the terminals and thus becomes stainable, or whether in old age and certain degenerative diseases the cell produces an abnormal substance. It remains to be seen whether this phenomenon is restricted to sheep or whether it also occurs in other species.

This work was supported by grants from the National Fund for Research into Crippling Diseases (to A. B.) and the National Foundation for Neuromuscular Diseases of New York (to H. B. P.).

[1] Beck, E., Daniel, P. M., and Parry, H. B., *Brain*, **87**, 153 (1964).
[2] Beck, E., Daniel, P. M., Gajdusek, D. C., and Gibbs, jun., C. J., in *Virus Diseases and the Nervous System*, 140 (Blackwell Scientific Publications, Oxford and Edinburgh, 1969).
[3] Parry, H. B., in *Virus Diseases and the Nervous System*, 99 (Blackwell Scientific Publications, Oxford and Edinburgh, 1969).
[4] Zambrano, D., and de Robertis, E. Z., *Z. Zellforsch.*, **81**, 264 (1967).
[5] Adams, C. W. M., and Sloper, J. C., *J. Endocrinol.*, **13**, 221 (1956).
[6] Sloper, J. C., *Nature*, **179**, 148 (1957).
[7] Hild, W., and Zetler, G., *Z. Ges. Exp. Med.*, **120**, 236 (1953).
[8] Sloper, J. C., in *The Pituitary Gland*, **3**, 131 (Butterworths, London, 1966).

THE FINE STRUCTURE OF NEUROFIBRILLARY TANGLES IN ALZHEIMER'S DISEASE † ‡

Robert D. Terry, M.D.§

The neurofibrillary tangle of Alzheimer is one of the most distinctive cytopathologic changes that occurs in the central nervous system. This communication presents the ultrastructure of neurofibrillary tangles as they were seen in brain biopsies of two patients with advanced Alzheimer's disease. The relation between these abnormal formations and certain other cell structures will be discussed.

MATERIAL AND METHODS

The biopsies§ are removed from the cerebral cortex at craniotomy. A wide region of bone is elevated and a dural flap turned on the non-dominant side. A gyrus is selected which is free of major vessels, and the leptomeninges are peeled off from a small area. A segment of cortex about 1 cm. square is quickly outlined with a pointed scalpel. This piece is scooped out, and only then are hemostatic measures applied. The biopsy, lying on a chilled polyethylene plate, is divided into three parts. The first slice is 1 to 2 mm. thick and is placed in formalin for light microscopy. The second portion is about 1 mm. thick and is flooded with buffered osmic acid (1) to which sucrose (2) has been added. The remainder (200 to 500 mgm.) of the biopsy is chilled for metabolic and chemical analyses (3). The tissue for electron microscopy is divided into blocks less than 1 mm. on each side, and fixation is continued for 90 minutes at 4°C. The blocks are then dehydrated in graded ethanol and embedded in methacrylate or Epon (4). The polymerized blocks are sectioned on a Porter-Blum microtome with glass or diamond knives, and the sections are mounted on Formvar or parlodion-covered copper grids. The contrast is enhanced by a lead hydroxide stain modified by Winkler from the technic of Millonig (5). A carbon film is then evaporated over the methacrylate sections. The electron micrographs are taken with a Siemens Elmiskop I.

CASE REPORTS

Case 1: This 62 year old woman entered the Neurological Service of the Bronx Municipal Hospital Center with a 7 year history of progressive dementia. During the 2 years prior to admission she became unable to care for herself, and was severely deteriorated.

The past history was otherwise irrelevant, and the family history was unknown.

The physical examination was unremarkable. The patient was agitated and displayed plucking motions of her hands, but was emotionally depressed. She was poorly oriented as to time and place, and was unable to recite the alphabet or to count. Language was markedly disrupted. Urinary incontinence was present. The cranial nerves functioned nor-

† This paper was presented in part at the Annual Meeting of the American Association of Neuropathologists, June 17, 1962.
‡ This study was supported by grants B-2255 and B-3356 from the National Institute of Neurological Diseases and Blindness.
§ I wish to thank the members of the Neurological and Neurosurgical Services for their cooperation in this study.

203

mally. The gait was shuffling, slow and hesitant. Myoclonic jerks were apparent in the upper extremities. The reflexes were normal.

The spinal fluid pressure was 104 mm H_2O. It contained no leukocytes. The protein was 46.5 mg per cent and the sugar was 78 mg. per cent. The electroencephalogram was diffusely abnormal.

A right sided parieto-occipital brain biopsy was performed. The postoperative course was characterized by steady deterioration of her mental status. Her increased aggressiveness caused her to be transferred to another hospital where she died several months after operation. Autopsy* confirmed the biopsy diagnosis of Alzheimer's presenile dementia.

Case 2: This 63 year old woman was admitted to the Neurological Service of the Bronx Municipal Hospital Center with a 1½ year history of progressive mental deterioration which was first noted when she became unable to sign her name. Shortly thereafter, memory loss became apparent. During the 18 months prior to admission, the patient frequently became lost in the street. She was unable to do her housework and had increasing difficulty in finding words.

The past history and family history were not informative.

The general physical and neurologic examination was normal. The patient did not know her name, her home address, the season of the year, or her location. Her recent memory was very poor, and she was not able to perform simple calculations or to recite the alphabet. Myoclonic jerks of the head, arms and trunk first appeared during hospitalization.

Severe cerebral atrophy was noted in a pneumoencephalogram. The electroencephalogram recorded frequent synchronous bursts of 3 to 4 *per* second activity. Spinal fluid protein was 27 mg per cent, sugar was 40 mg per cent and there were 5 leukocytes.

A biopsy was made of the second right frontal convolution. The patient tolerated the operative procedure well and was later transferred to a state mental hospital.

GROSS EXAMINATION AND LIGHT MICROSCOPY

Case 1: Although the gyrus was slightly narrower than usual, the cortical ribbon was not abnormally thinned. The tissue was firm to the knife. Microscopically, the cortical architecture was well preserved although there was mild gliosis. Neuronal loss was very slight. Bodian stains revealed many neurofibrillary tangles and a moderate number of senile plaques (fig. 1). The former were made up of rather delicate intraneuronal fibers. The plaques did not have the typical central core of amorphous material, but were composed of loosely organized aggregates of irregular clubs and thick fibers lying in a clear matrix which appeared to be extracellular space.

Case 2: In this biopsy, the cortex was seen to be moderately thinner than normal. Microscopic examination demonstrated a mild loss of neurons. The layers of the cortex were normally distinct. Bodian preparations showed numerous neurofibrillary tangles similar to those of the first case. Senile plaques were not found.

ELECTRON MICROSCOPY

The over-all image of cortical organization was unremarkable. The neuropil was close-packed and made up of great numbers of cell processes of varying diameter and density. Extracellular space was generally limited to the gap between apposed cell membranes, and measured about 200 Å in width. A few

* The author is grateful to Dr. Irwin Feigin, Professor of Neuropathology, College of Medicine, New York University, for having made this information available.

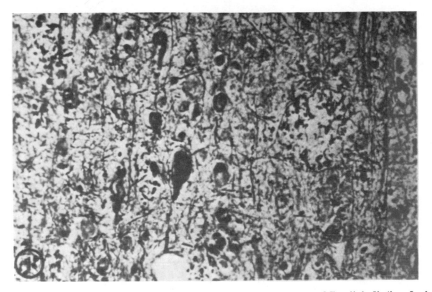

Symbols used on electron micrographs: *G*, Golgi apparatus; *GF*, glial fibrils; *L*, lysosome; *LA*, lipid aggregate; *LP*, lipofuscin; *M*, mitochondrion; *N*, Nissl substance; *NF*, neurofilaments; *S*, synapse

Fig. 1. Bodian preparation of cortex in Case I. The neurofibrillary tangles and the senile plaques are displayed. × 310.

larger and more irregular intercellular spaces sometimes occurred between the corners of adjacent processes. There was no recognizable material, either fibrillar or particulate, in these extracellular regions.

All plasma membranes were distinct and of the usual thickness. There was no evidence of any abnormal deposits on either their internal or external surfaces.

Most neurons were normal (figs. 2, 3). Their nucleoplasm was finely divided and quite regularly dispersed, although there was a slight tendency to flocculation of the nuclear granules toward the periphery. The nucleoli were compact, but not entirely solid, aggregates of somewhat coarser granules. The nuclear membrane was double. Not infrequently the two membrane profiles were seen to join and form a single, thin layer which for a short distance was the only separation between nucleoplasm and cytoplasm. These were the nuclear pores. Less commonly, the outer nuclear membrane was visibly continuous with the granulated endoplasmic reticulum.

The concentration of ergastoplasm varied very considerably from one neuron to another. Clusters and rosettes of 150 Å granules were prominent among the flat sacs of ergastoplasm. Golgi apparatus was an important component of the neuronal cytoplasm and consisted of clusters of vesicles and flattened sacs. The Golgi aggregates were found most often close to the nucleus, but also in occasional sites throughout the perikaryon and in the major dendrites.

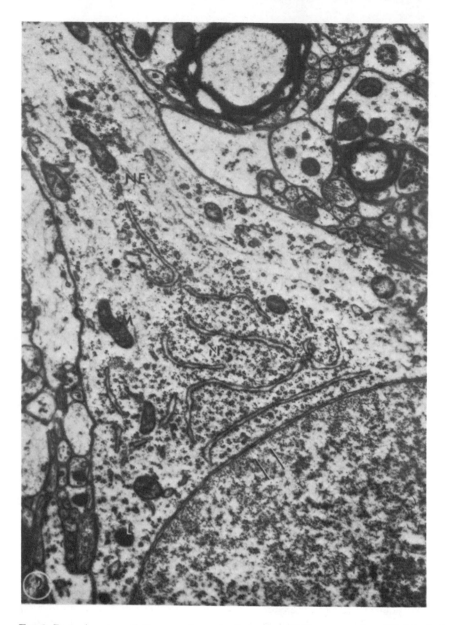

FIG. 2. Part of an essentially normal neuron from Case 2. The paranuclear Nissl body is clear because there is little other basophilic material nearby. Sparse neurofilaments, mitochondria and a few lysosomes are present. Nuclear pores are evident at the arrows. The neuropil is compact. Adjacent myelin is artefactitiously ruffled; × 18,000.

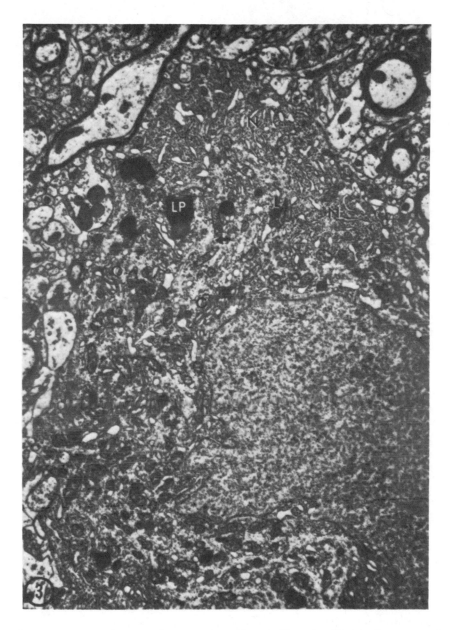

Fig. 3. An essentially normal neuron from Case 2. Here the Nissl bodies are poorly demarcated. Golgi apparatus, mitochondria and lysosomes are abundant. A few neurofibrils (*arrow*) are present in the hyaloplasm. Several lipofuscin bodies are visible; × 9,200.

Lipofuscin granules were quite common and had a characteristic, compound appearance. They were rounded but irregular, and were closely surrounded by a single membrane. Most of the lipid body was very dense, but there was usually a smoothly contoured region of lesser density and remarkable homogeneity. Occasional coarse granules and short membranes could sometimes be distinguished in the denser zone. Lysosome-like dense bodies were also found scattered at random. These organelles measured about 0.34 μ in diameter in these human neurons, were generally round, and were bounded by a single membrane. They were filled by fine, evenly dispersed granules of moderate density. These bodies were not apparently altered in the diseased neurons except for being displaced. However, among some aggregates of lipofuscin, there were moderately large and irregular organelles with the density of the lysosome-like bodies and the shape of lipofuscin.

Mitochondria were distributed at random in the cytoplasm. In the normal neurons their matrix was usually moderately dense, but in general it was not as dark as the mitochondrial matrix found in immediately adjacent neuropil elements. The mitochondria in neurons marked by neurofibrillary change were usually swollen and watery. They were in sharp contrast to normally dense mitochondria of other cells which were only a fraction of one micron distant.

Many neurons displayed abnormally prominent neurofibrils. These were distributed in the neuronal cytoplasm in 3 ways. The most common arrangement was as small bundles, 0.5 to 1.0 μ wide, of loosely aggregated, roughly aligned fibrils (figs. 4, 5). Sometimes these bundles were considerably wider and occupied much of the perikaryon (figs. 6, 7). The least common distribution was as a more uniform and less close-packed dispersal of neurofilaments throughout much of the cytoplasm (fig. 8). Among these latter fibrils were normal organelles. Intermediate in frequency was a very dense, broad group of oriented fibrils which completely filled one end of a cell. Here the normal organelles and hyaloplasm were almost entirely displaced (fig. 9).

The individual neurofibrils were essentially similar in all of these situations. Their true length was not measurable because of the thinness of the sections, but was in the order of several microns. Their width was found to vary around a mean of 100 Å. The narrowest were 70 Å wide and the thickest about 125 Å. They displayed a tubule-like triple density, with pale center and dense borders. The central zone was usually slightly wider than the edge. The density of the fibrils was somewhat less than that of cell membranes or of ribosomes. The neurofilaments did not branch, nor did they anastomose with one another (fig. 10).

The fibrils were not spatially related to other intraneuronal cytoplasmic organelles in any regular way. Continuity between endoplasmic reticulum and neurofibrils was not demonstrated. Some neurons with large concentrations of lipofuscin granules showed severe neurofibrillary change, while in other cells tangles of filaments were prominent and there was no lipofuscin. Large, close-packed groups of fibrils often displaced other organelles, but there was some tendency to spare small groups of Golgi sacs and vesicles.

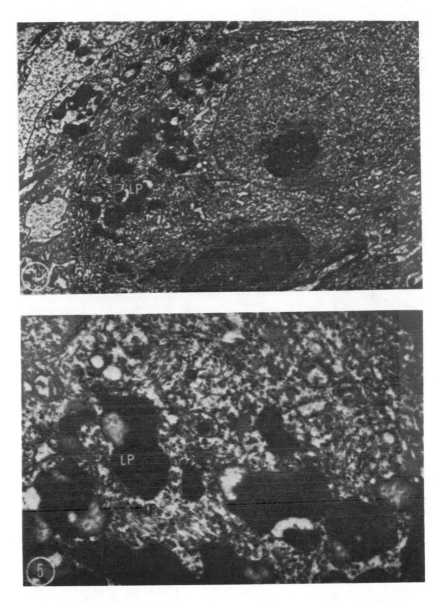

Fig. 4. A moderately affected neuron from Case 1. A small satellite cell with dense cytoplasm lies below the large neuron. Between the lipofuscin bodies there are many bundles of neurofibrils (arrows). × 6,800.

Fig. 5. A higher magnification of part of the previous picture emphasizes the neurofibrils. The single membrane bounding lipofuscin is visible; × 20,000.

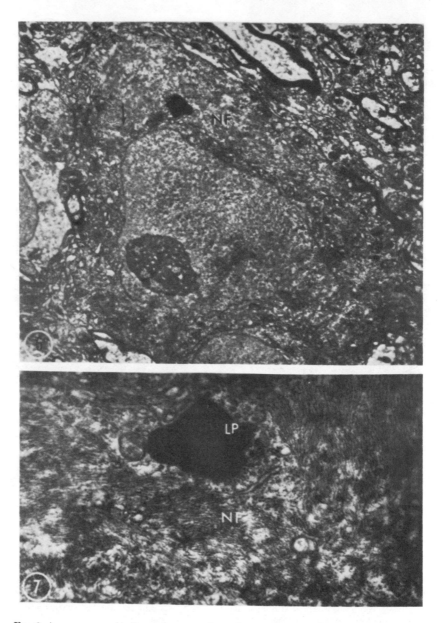

FIG. 6. A more severely diseased neuron from Case 2. Wide bundles of neurofilaments fill much of the cytoplasm. The neuronal mitochrondria are swollen and watery compared with those outside. A so-called spine apparatus is present in the perikaryon at the arrow; × 8,600.
FIG. 7. A higher magnification of part of Figure 6; × 29,000.

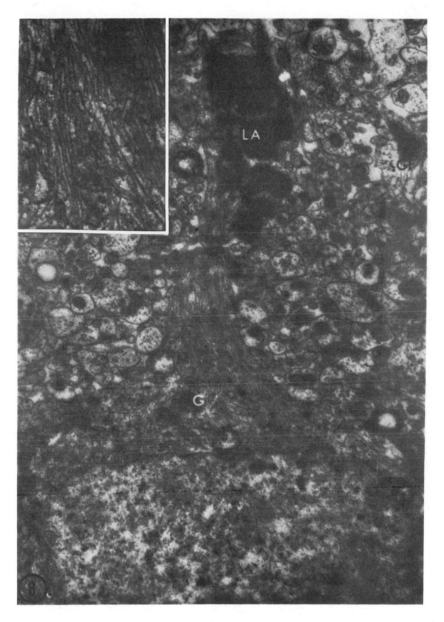

Fig. 8. A neuron from Case 2 with evenly dispersed neurofibrils running out into a dendrite. Lipid material distends part of the dendrite to form a torpedo; × 14,000. The inset shows the triple density of the neurofilaments; × 42,000.

211

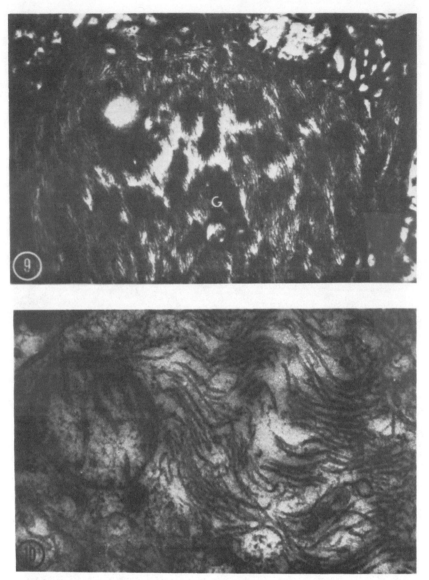

Fig. 9. One end of a neuron from Case 2. This portion of the perikaryon is completely filled by neurofilaments. All organelles are displaced except some of the Golgi apparatus; × 22,000.

Fig. 10. Perikaryon neurofilaments of Case 2. Their tubular character is apparent; × 57,000.

A variable and moderate degree of gliosis was apparent in the cortex. This was evidenced by long cell processes with relatively clear hyaloplasm containing many loosely arranged, solid fibrils which were 60 to 70 Å wide. These glial fibrils were never seen without surrounding cytoplasm and plasma membrane.

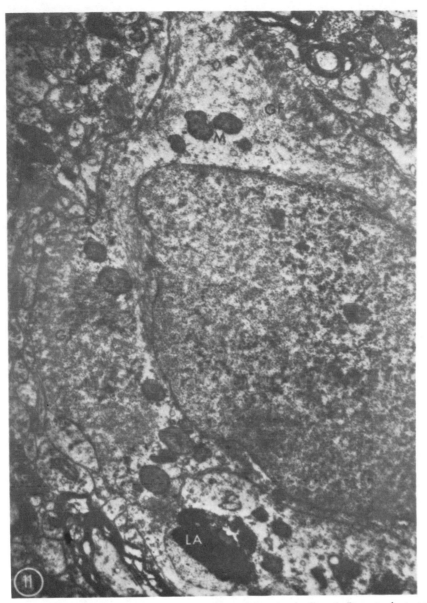

Fig. 11. A hypertrophied, fibrous astrocyte from the cortex in Case 1. Its cytoplasm contains many delicate fibrils. The mitochondria are poor in cristae. Endoplasmic reticulum is sparse. The neuropil is compact; × 15,000.

Mitochondria were often present next to the fibrils in these cellular extensions. These fibril-containing cells correspond to the astrocytes of classical neurocytology. The cell bodies of these glia were enlarged and often rounded (fig. 11). The hyaloplasm was light and surrounded large numbers of delicate fibrils similar to those in the more distant glial processes. Ergastoplasm and Golgi apparatus were sparse, while the mitochondria were moderately numerous. These had dense, granular matrix and few cristae.

DISCUSSION

Although many descriptions of the ultrastructure of axonal and dendritic neurofibrils have been published, there is a remarkable paucity of detail concerning these elements in the perikaryon. Several times their very existence at the fine structure level has been denied, or has been suggested to be artefactual (6–8). Palay and Palade (9), however, did note occasional bundles of fibrils, 60 to 100 Å wide, coursing through the cytoplasm between clumps of Nissl substance. Roizin and Dmochowski (10) saw individual fibrils but did not measure them, while Schultz, Maynard and Pease (11) mentioned filaments 100 to 200 Å wide. The hypertrophic sensory ganglion cells of the lizard contain numerous 60 to 70 Å wide solid fibrils (12). Filaments in the perikaryon or in the axon have been described as solid, while dendritic neurofibrils measure 200 Å, and have been repeatedly found to be tubular. More recently Palay has noted that the 100 Å wide fibrils within the neuronal cell bodies are also hollow (13). The abnormally prominent neurofibrils of Alzheimer's disease are thus apparently not different in structure from those of the normal cell body.

At most, neurofilaments are very sparse in the normal neuronal perikaryon. A clear difference in fibril concentration exists between the normal neurons described elsewhere and many of the neurons from the two biopsies reported here. But there is a spectrum of fibril concentration from a normal number to a complete replacement of cytoplasm in the diseased cortex.

Artefacts of hydration, such as expanded ergastoplasmic sacs, are almost inevitable, to at least a minor degree, in tissue taken under such complex circumstances as those which obtain at human craniotomy, and fixed by immersion rather than by perfusion. Although fibril formation as the result of this sort of artefact is unknown, mitochondrial swelling is very common in all sorts of tissue. Furthermore, neuronal mitochondria are often less dense than those seen elsewhere. But the distribution of swollen mitochondria in these biopsies is strikingly confined to diseased neurons while mitochondria in adjacent glia, less than one micron distant, are of normal size and density as are those in normal neurons. Specific swelling of neuronal mitochondria is not unique for Alzheimer's disease in that a similar discrete phenomenon has been noted in Jakob-Creutzfeldt disease (14). This alteration of neuronal mitochondria seems to be more than a simple artefact. It may reflect a lessened reserve in the diseased neurons of some very rapidly utilized substrate such as glucose or oxygen.

The extracellular space in these cortical biopsies, is limited to a gap of 100 to 200 Å, which is within normal limits. Syneresis has been evoked as a causal process in this disease, but evidence for it is lacking in the current study.

The absence in these tissues of extracellular neurofibrillary tangles has several possible explanations: (1) extracellular tangles do not exist except as artefacts produced by the preparative methods used for light microscopy; (2) neither patient had deteriorated to the stage where the neurons disintegrate in the frontal cortex; (3) the restricted samples did not happen to include these degenerative forms. Extraneuronal tangles are most common in the Ammon's horn of the hippocampus. In view of their rarity in the frontal cortex, the third explanation seems most likely but there is no conclusive proof of this. A similar explanation may be extended to our failure to find senile plaques in the electronmicroscopic studies although they were visible in Bodian preparations of the first specimen. Another possibility, however, is that the plaques were simply not recognized. The fact that tangles look just as might have been expected on the basis of our previous experience need not indicate that the plaques would also have a familiar shape and density.

The theory of Divry (15) concerning the relationship of amyloid to the neurofibrillary change of Alzheimer becomes more interesting in the light of recent electron microscopic studies of experimental amyloidosis (16–18). All such analyses have found amyloid to be, at least in part, a fibrillar protein with the elements lying in oriented bundles. Most of these fascicles lie in the extracellular space, but a few are found within the cytoplasm of reticulo-endothelial cells. The fibrils are reported by some to be 100 Å thick, while other investigators have measured their width as only 50 Å. There is also dispute as to whether the amyloid fibrils are solid or tubular. Aside from their common staining properties, there is some structural basis for a comparison between amyloid and neurofibrillary tangles.

On the basis of extensive physical and chemical studies (19) involving chiefly invertebrate axoplasm, Schmitt and Davison have proposed that neurofibrils are 100 Å wide tubules made up of helically wound protofibrils, each composed of chains of globular protein molecules. The correspondence between this hypothetical diagram and the demonstrated perikaryon neurofibril is striking.

SUMMARY

1. Electron microscopic studies of two cortical biopsies in Alzheimer's disease are reported.

2. Neurofibrillary tangles were made of bundles of 100 Å hollow fibrils occupying the neuronal cytoplasm and displacing the normal organelles.

3. In the affected neurons the mitochondria were swollen and watery.

4. The neuropil was normal save for moderate gliosis. The long glial processes contained solid 60 Å fibrils.

5. Neurofibrillary tangles and glial fibrils were never seen except inside cells.

6. The hyopthetical neurofibril diagram of Schmitt and Davison is noted to be remarkably similar to the electron micrographs of filaments in both normal and diseased human neurons.

Acknowledgment: The skilled technical assistance of Martin Weiss, M.A. and of Robin Winkler, B.A. is gratefully acknowledged. I also wish to thank Dr. S. R. Korey and Dr. A. A. Angrist for their advice and comments.

REFERENCES

1. PALADE, G. E.: The Fixation of Tissues for Electron Microscopy. J. Exper. Med., 95: 285, 1952.
2. CAULFIELD, J. B.: Effect of Varying the Vehicle for OsO₄ in Tissue Fixation. J. Biophys. Biochem. Cytol., 3: 827, 1957.
3. KOREY, S. R.: To be published.
4. LUFT, J. H.: Improvements in Epoxy Embedding Methods. J. Biophys. Biochem. Cytol., 9: 409, 1961.
5. MILLONIG, G.: A Modified Procedure for Lead Staining of Thin Sections. J. Biophys. Biochem. Cytol., 11: 736, 1961.
6. PEASE, D. C., AND BAKER, R. F.: Electron Microscopy of Nervous Tissue. Anat. Record, 110: 505, 1951.
7. HONJIN, R.: Electron Microscopy of Peripheral Nerve Fibers. Folia Anat. Jap., 27: 179, 1955.
8. SCHARRER, E., AND BROWN, S.: Neurosecretion. XII. The Formation of Neurosecretory Granules in the Earthworm, Lumbricus Terrestris L. Ztschr. f. Zellforsch., 54: 530, 1961.
9. PALAY, S. L., AND PALADE, G. E.: The Fine Structure of Neurons. J. Biophys. Biochem. Cytol., 1: 69, 1955.
10. ROIZIN, L., AND DMOCHOWSKY, L.: Comparative Histologic and Electron Microscope Investigations of the Central Nervous System. J. Neuropath. & Exper. Neurol., 15: 12, 1956.
11. SCHULTZ, R. L., MAYNARD, E. A., AND PEASE, D. C.: Electron Microscopy of Neurons and Neuroglia of Cerebral Cortex and Corpus Callosum. Am. J. Anat., 100: 369, 1957.
12. PANNESE, E.: Detection of Neurofilaments in the Perikaryon of Hypertrophic Nerve Cells. J. Cell Biol., 13: 457, 1962.
13. PALAY, S. L.: Neuronal Ultrastructure. In Macromolecular Specificity in Biological Membranes, F. O. Schmitt, Ed., Cambridge, M.I.T. Press, 1962.
14. GONATAS, N. K., AND TERRY, R. D.: To be published.
15. DIVRY, P.: De la Nature de l'Alteration Fibrillaire d'Alzheimer. J. Belge de Neurol. et Psychiat., 34: 197, 1934.
16. COHEN, A. S., AND CALKINS, E.: Electron Microscopic Observations on a Fibrous Component in Amyloid of Diverse Origins. Nature, 183: 1202, 1959.
17. GHIDONI, J., AND GUEFT, B.: The Double Nature of the Amyloid Fibril. Proc. Fifth Internat. Cong. for Elect. Mic., p. T-15, New York, Academic Press, 1962.
18. HEEFNER, W. A., AND SORENSON, G. D.: Experimental Amyloidosis I. Light and Electron Microscopic Observations of Spleen and Lymph Nodes. Lab. Invest., 11: 585, 1962.
19. SCHMITT, F. O., AND DAVIDSON, P. F.: Biologie Moléculaire des Neurofilaments. In Actualités Neurophysiologiques, Y.M. Monnier, Ed., Paris, Masson, 1962.

ULTRASTRUCTURAL STUDIES IN ALZHEIMER'S PRESENILE DEMENTIA

Robert D. Terry, M.D.; Nicholas K. Gonatas, M.D.,
and Martin Weiss, M.A.

An electron microscopic study of cerebral biopsy specimens from 3 cases of Alzheimer's presenile dementia has revealed several points of interest. The two major findings have to do with the neurofibrillary tangles and senile plaques which are the characteristic features of this disease. It will be shown that the former are made up of large clusters of fine neurofibrils, while plaques have as their fundamental substance a different sort of filamentous material which is structurally identical to amyloid. Also noteworthy are certain myelin distortions suggestive of primary demyelinization; and a striking, although rare, endothelial change by which lipid-like material passes through the walls of small vessels to enter the lumen.

Case Histories and Light Microscopy

Case 1

A 62-year-old woman had a 7-year history of slowly progressive dementia. During the 1½ years prior to admission, she was unable to care for herself, and required nursing attention. A coarse, shaking tremor was attributed to Parkinsonism. The family history was not known.

The general physical examination was unremarkable. The patient was agitated, depressed and poorly oriented. She could not carry out simple commands, recite the alphabet or count. There were myoclonic jerks of the upper extremities. The gait was hesitant and shuffling. The face was mask-like and there was a questionable intention tremor. Muscle tone was not increased. An electroencephalogram showed a diffusely abnormal tracing. The spinal fluid protein was 47 mg. per cent, but the fluid was not otherwise remarkable. Other laboratory examinations were not unusual.

A biopsy specimen was procured from the right parieto-occipital region at craniotomy. Mental deterioration continued during the weeks after operation. Many months after operation the patient died at another hospital. Necropsy confirmed the biopsy diagnosis.

The cerebral cortex of the biopsy specimen was slightly thinner and tougher than normal. The cortical architecture was well preserved microscopically and there was only minimal gliosis. Bodian preparations revealed numerous intraneuronal, coarse neurofibrillary tangles. Many senile plaques were also found. They were composed of argentophilic fibers and granules. Core material was poorly demonstrated. The pathologic diagnosis was Alzheimer's presenile dementia.

Supported by Grants NB-02255 and NB-03356 from the National Institute of Neurological Diseases and Blindness, National Institutes of Health, United States Public Health Service.

Case 2

A 63-year-old woman had a 1½-year history of progressive dementia beginning with inability to sign her name properly. She became particularly forgetful, got lost frequently and had difficulty in word-finding and in caring for herself. The past history and family history were not contributory.

The general physical and neurologic examinations were normal except for myoclonic jerks of the head, arms and trunk. She was fearful, disoriented and apraxic. Her memory span was very short and she was unable to perform simple calculations or to recite the alphabet. An electroencephalogram exhibited a diffusely abnormal pattern. A pneumoencephalogram revealed marked cortical atrophy.

A biopsy of the second right frontal gyrus was made at craniotomy. The patient quickly resumed her pre-operative state, and was later discharged to a state psychiatric hospital.

The cortex was thin and the leptomeninges moderately thickened. Bodian preparations showed many neurofibrillary tangles. Senile plaques could not be demonstrated. There was mild neuronal loss. Gliosis was slight in both cortex and white matter. The pathologic diagnosis was Alzheimer's presenile dementia.

Case 3

A 52-year-old woman had a 3-year history of progressive memory loss and increasingly repetitive speech. She became unable to do her housework and required nursing care at home during the 15 months prior to admission. There was a history of proven and suspected Alzheimer's disease among several relatives on the maternal side and 3 of 4 siblings.

The physical examination was not contributory. The affect was inappropriate and labile. Severe loss of recent memory, very short attention span and marked expressive aphasia were noted. The gait was broad-based. Muscle tone was uniformly increased, and there was suggestive cog-wheel rigidity at the wrists and elbows. Reflexes were normal. Sensory examination was not possible. An electroencephalogram exhibited a mild, diffusely abnormal pattern, but all other laboratory tests were unremarkable.

Biopsy was made in the second right prefontal gyrus at craniotomy. Following a short period of confusion and low fever, the patient returned to her pre-operative state and was later discharged to another institution. She died several months later, and necropsy confirmed the diagnosis which had been made on the biopsy specimen.

The cortex in the specimen was thin and exhibited moderate gliosis. The cortical layers were still apparent, but the architecture was not well preserved. Neurofibrillary tangles were rare and not very dense. There were, however, many senile plaques, which were seen as circular zones of very finely granular material with a few argentophilic rods, fibers and granules. Microglial nuclei were prominent within these plaques. The remaining neurons contained much lipofuscin which stained in positive manner with the periodic acid-Schiff and Sudan IV stains. The diagnosis was Alzheimer's disease.

Methods

The procedures have been detailed previously [1] and need only be summarized here. The biopsy specimen was removed from the nondominant hemisphere at craniotomy where a full-sized bone flap was turned. Hemostasis was secured only after removal of the tissue. The specimen weighed less than 1 gm., and was quickly divided into 3 portions. That for light microscopy was fixed in cold formalin. Bodian, Heidenhain, gallocyanin, Congo red, and periodic acid-Schiff stains were carried out on paraffin-embedded material. Sudan, Spielmeyer, acid phosphatase [2,3] and thiamine pyrophosphatase [4] preparations were made from frozen sections. The last two were for the purpose of demonstrating lysosomes and Golgi apparatus respectively. Tissue for chemical and metabolic studies (results to be reported elsewhere) was chilled in Tris

218

buffer. The material for electron microscopy was fixed in veronal-buffered osmic acid [5] with sucrose,[6] dehydrated in alcohol and embedded in methacrylate, Epon [7] and Araldite.[8] The thin sections were stained with lead hydroxide [9] alone or in combination with uranyl acetate.[10] The electron micrographs were taken with a Siemens Elmiskop I. The studies were based on examination of 152 blocks of tissue. More than 1,300 micrographs were made.

ELECTRON MICROSCOPY

Plaques

The senile plaque of Alzheimer's disease as seen with the electron microscope, had 4 major components: (a) central fibrillar core; (b) cellular perikarya; (c) axons and dendrites filled with an excess of neurofibrils; (d) cell processes filled with dense bodies.

The central core of the plaque was a stellate mass (Figs. 1 to 5) of interwoven fibrils, each 70 to 90 Å wide. The individual fibrils (Fig. 6) had a triple density indicating a hollow center. The light, central portion was about ⅓ the total thickness. Periodicity in the longitudinal dimension was lacking. There were no formed elements between the fibrils, nor was there a ground substance of appreciable density. The fibrils were often grouped into bundles, but there were no membranes segregating these bundles and, furthermore, single fibrils often passed from one bundle to the next in both cross and longitudinal sections. There was a tendency to directional orientation of the fibrils within many bundles, but this was imperfect as indicated by their interweaving. In addition, some orientation of the bundles was noted; they generally radiated outward from the center of the plaque. Collagen was not present.

While the central fibrils and bundles were clearly extracellular (Figs. 5 and 6), those toward the periphery of the plaque were found in intimate relationship to nuclei and cellular organelles. The involved cells had deeply and irregularly indented borders facing the central core. Masses of the extracellular fibrils fitted loosely into these indentations, but were, in these regions, separated from intracellular material by the plasma membrane (Fig. 7). They were at times within 200 mμ of the nuclear membrane. The convoluted plasma membrane in these areas was often unsharp and incomplete.

Bundles of fibrils appeared less commonly to be intracytoplasmic and to be without any direct continuity with extracellular material (Figs. 8 and 9). These cells had elongated, irregular nuclei, very similar to those of the cells involved as described above. The cytoplasm contained moderate numbers of free ribosomes and was usually of medium density. There was little ergastoplasm. The bundles of poorly oriented fibrils dominated a portion of the cell body. A boundary membrane only partly surrounded the bundles. In some areas the fibrils seemed not to

219

be separated from the cytoplasm. Continuities with the membranes of ergastoplasm or the Golgi apparatus could not be distinguished.

Many enlarged axons and dendrites (Fig. 10) containing abnormal numbers of neurofilaments were arranged in a haphazard fashion about the periphery of the core of the plaque. These filaments were closely packed within the neuronal processes, with some tendency to spare that part of the cytoplasm immediately under the plasma membrane. The long axis of most of the neurofibrils lay in the long axis of the cell process, but some took a spiral course. The filaments varied in diameter from 100 to 200 Å, and in some regions appeared to be twisted at irregular intervals of 30 to several hundred mμ (Figs. 11 and 12). They were of the same appearance whether in myelinated or unmyelinated processes.

In many of the neuronal processes there were variable numbers of small, round, dense bodies (Figs. 1 to 4 and 13). These measured about 0.5 μ, with a diameter range of 0.3 to 1.0 μ. They were much more common in unmyelinated processes than in sheathed axons. When there were only a few of the dense bodies, they were found at the periphery of the process, while groups of neurofilaments filled most of it. However, many dendrites were nearly filled by dozens of these small bodies. Between them there were usually a few filaments, which still permitted the cell processes to be identified as neuronal extensions. These swollen dendrites or axons were most common in and around the plaques where they occurred in clusters. Scattered throughout the cortex were occasional single dendrites containing similar organelles. It was apparent at higher magnification that the dense bodies were at least partly composed of membranes. A few thin layers often surrounded a more homogeneous, very dark core. Less commonly the bodies were made up of many membranes, which sometimes displayed a very considerable regularity of spacing. This periodicity varied widely between 45 and 100 Å.

There were moderately increased numbers of glial cell processes at the periphery of the plaque and to a lesser extent throughout the cortex. The glial cellular extensions contained loose clusters of non-interwoven, solid fibrils which were 60 to 70 Å wide. The astrocyte perikarya were moderately enlarged and also contained groups of similar fibrils (Fig. 14). Glial fibrils were not found outside a plasma membrane. The astrocytes often contained lipid aggregates closely resembling lipofuscin but usually with several small vacuoles in the less dense component.

Neurofibrillary Change of Alzheimer

Our observations relating to the neurofibrillary tangles in the first 2 cases have already been reported.[11] Case 3 has added more data, but has not changed the conclusions. The tangles, therefore, will be treated only briefly here.

In the thin sections used for electron microscopy, neurofibrils were quite sparse within normal neuronal perikarya. The fibrils were of two general types: those measuring about 100 Å (90 to 125 Å) in width and resembling axonal filaments, and those about 200 Å (180 to 210 Å) wide and resembling dendritic tubules. Both types (Figs. 11 and 12) had a triple density as seen in longitudinal section, with dense edges and light cores. Some seemed to twist, in that they were intermittently narrowed. In cross section the neurofilaments were occasionally found as circlets, but were more often seen as short, curved elements with the familiar dense-light-dense structure. They were essentially similar to the filaments found within neuronal processes involved in senile plaques.

Neurofibrillary tangles were made up of similar elements which were present in greatly increased numbers and were arranged in large bundles (Figs. 15 and 16). There was little or no interweaving among the neurofilaments within a bundle. These groups of fibrils often occupied the greater portion of the neuronal cytoplasm and displaced the mitochondria, lysosomes, ergastoplasm and Golgi apparatus (Figs. 17 and 18). The filaments within a bundle were quite uniformly oriented, and were for the most part of the 100 Å variety. Continuities between the filaments and the normal cellular organelles were not found.

Many lipofuscin bodies (Fig. 19) were present in most large neurons, but the amount of lipofuscin could not be correlated either negatively or positively with abnormal neurofibrillary bundles. The lipofuscin was composed of dense, homogeneous, granular or membranous material closely associated with lighter, very homogeneous matter. A unit membrane surrounded each of these compound bodies.

Myelin

Large numbers of widely scattered, abnormal axons were manifest. In many of these, the axoplasm itself was morphologically intact. It displayed its usual filamentous material, mitochondria and light hyaloplasm, and it was bounded by a continuous axolemma. The myelin surrounding these apparently normal axis cylinders, however, was interrupted, bubbled and granular (Figs. 20 to 22). The lamellas were not simply spread apart and ruffled, as is seen when embedding artifacts occur. Rather, there were wide zones between lamellas, filled with dense, granular debris and small vacuoles, the latter enclosed by two or more membranes with a spacing which approximated half that of normal myelin. The granular material had a density similar to that of the major period line of myelin. These damaged areas were found in either deep or superficial regions of the sheath, and were noted for the most part in sheaths of at least medium thickness. The lamellar destruction did not usually involve the full thickness of the myelin. It more often spared a few layers on the outside and a few adjacent to the axolemma. Nevertheless, there was unquestionable loss of myelin lamellas in these granular zones, since the total number of remaining lamellas inside the zone plus those outside the zone was less than the number of myelin layers elsewhere around the circumference of the axon.

Quite another form of axonal abnormality had essentially normal myelin while the axis cylinder filled only a small portion of the cross-section area. The rest of this space was taken up with one or a few large vacuoles (Fig. 23). These were bounded by a double membrane which had no clear connection with the myelin, and they contained only very little granular material. One layer of the double boundary membrane was sometimes broken and appeared to end in a ball or knot. The origin of these membranes or of the vacuolar contents remained uncertain. They compressed the axis cylinder into an irregular polyhedron which was not otherwise remarkable.

In a few instances, the myelin sheath was intact while the axoplasm was dense and granular. Late forms of axonal degeneration were also found. Digestion chambers and myelin whorls similar to those of wallerian degeneration [12,13] were noted (Fig. 24) in cortex and white matter. The normal myelin period of about 120 Å was maintained well after the sheath lost its continuity.

Only the superficial white matter was available for study. A moderate increase in extracellular space was noted, but it could not be determined whether this was the result of imperfect preparative methods or of a pathologic alteration. Occasional glial processes here and in the cortex contained dense lipid aggregates which were partially laminated (Fig. 25). A few of these resembled the membranous cytoplasmic bodies (Fig. 26) of Tay-Sachs disease.[14]

Vessels

Most vessels appeared to be quite normal. There were, however, numerous perithelial cells containing lipid droplets (Fig. 27). These cells were separated from the adjacent parenchyma by a basement membrane, the thickness of which varied widely. The lipid droplets contained both very dense and relatively light material. A unit membrane separated the lipid from the surrounding cytoplasm.

The endothelial cells occasionally contained lipid droplets similar to those of the perithelium. Also present here were small, irregularly outlined aggregates of closely packed, dense granules (Fig. 28). An intimate unit membrane could sometimes be distinguished at the edge of the aggregate. This dense material was often just under the lumen plasma membrane. In a few instances the membrane was lost over a distance of 100 to 200 mμ, and the dense material, unbounded, lay in the gap extending into the adjacent lumen (Fig. 29).

A clearly related phenomenon was found with about the same frequency. In these instances, the inner (lumen) membrane was invaginated into the lumen where it formed a sphere 200 to 400 mμ in diameter (Fig. 30). It was connected to the endothelium by a narrow neck 50 to 100 mμ wide. An aggregate of the same dense, particulate material almost filled the sphere and the neck. The aggregate itself had its own unit membrane. In the lumen near the wall were occasional stemless vesicles and numerous irregular and unbounded dense aggregates which were less compact at their edges (Fig. 28).

Yet another vascular alteration was an occasional separation of the endothelial cells leaving a gap in the vascular lining so that basement membrane came into contact with lumen (Fig. 31). Residua of the cement line were apparent in the thickening of the facing endothelial plasma membranes, but an oblique fenestration up to 200 mμ wide separated these normally joined faces. Within the gap were several ovoid vesicles, each surrounded by a unit membrane. The vesicular contents varied in density but did not resemble cytoplasm. The vesicles were small, dense and indistinct within the somewhat widened, underlying basement membrane. Those nearer the lumen were larger and clearer.

The vascular abnormalities which have been described occurred primarily in thin-walled vessels 10 to 20 μ wide. They were either venules or large capillaries. The affected vessels were not scattered at random throughout the tissue but, rather, were found in several restricted areas.

DISCUSSION

Certain differences and similarities among the pathologic elements of Alzheimer's disease may now be summarized before their implications are discussed. Plaques and tangles have many features in common, but are structurally related in a very incomplete fashion. The filamentous material of the core of the plaque is quite different from that in the tangle. The cellular elements of the plaque are probably microglial, and are also independent of the tangle. On the other hand, the enlarged dendrites and axons of the plaques are filled with neurofilaments much as are the neuronal perikarya involved in Alzheimer's change. Dendritic or axonal dense bodies are prominent in the plaque and are of neuronal origin, but are not found in the tangle.

The 4 types of filaments found in this tissue may also be enumerated: (1) Neurofilaments 100 Å wide are found in axons and are common in neurofibrillary tangles and in abnormal dendrites. (2) Neurofilaments 200 Å wide are found in dendrites and are less common in the neuronal perikaryon. (3) Astrocytic fibrils are 60 Å wide and are solid as opposed to neurofilaments, both types of which are hollow. (4) Plaque fibrils are 90 Å wide, are interwoven and are also hollow.

The nature of senile and presenile brain changes has been much discussed. The classic concepts as well as certain histochemical information were presented in detail by Margolis.[15] The data dominating the classic concepts concerned largely the argentophilic and congophilic properties of the pathologic elements. The current ultrastructural studies permit clarification of some of the problems attending these complex phenomena.

It was Divry[16] who first noted that the senile plaque had staining reactions similar to those of amyloid. Divry and Florkin had previously suggested[17] that extraneural amyloid had a crystalloid structure despite its hyaline appearance. Recent electron microscopic studies by several groups of investigators[18-21] have demonstrated that this substance is composed of bundles of fine fibrils, but estimates of fiber diameter have varied widely from 50 to 300 Å. Ghidoni and Gueft[19] first described the hollow nature of the filament.

There is a remarkable correspondence between the image of experimentally induced splenic amyloidosis[20] and the core of the human senile plaque. The fibrils are similar; their rough orientation in bundles is similar; the stellate outline of the aggregate is similar. The combined evidence of fine structure, stain reactions and optical quality (birefringence) is so strong that we cannot doubt the identification of the core of the plaque as amyloid.

The source of this substance is uncertain, but it seems probable that it is a local cellular product, rather than a secretion from the blood. Heefner and Sorenson[20] have clearly demonstrated bundles of amyloid fibrils within the cytoplasm of splenic reticuloendothelial cells. The absence of a membrane surrounding these intracellular bundles makes it very unlikely that they have been phagocytosed. Cells in the senile plaque also contain these fibrils in their cytoplasm. The microglial cell is the counterpart in the central nervous system of the reticuloendothelial cell, and is very likely the source of amyloid material in the senile plaque. The question remains as to what stimulates these cells to produce this remarkable substance. Perhaps the stimulus comes from the abnormal neuronal components discussed below.

The aggregates of dense bodies found prominently within plaques are of unknown source and significance. Hydrated phospholipids are implicated by the structure of the membranous components. The variable periodicity and the irregular densities suggest that the chemical composition is inconstant. These bodies might be expected to stain positively with the periodic acid-Schiff reaction and variably with Sudan type reagents. They are distinct from the lipofuscin bodies which are found within neuronal perikarya. The latter are probably derived from lysosomes [22] and contain acid phosphatase.[23] Webster [24] has studied the early stages of wallerian degeneration in peripheral nerve and has noted focal accumulations of very similar dense bodies in distended axons distal to the experimental crush injury. He believed that they were derived from mitochondria. Regardless of their source, their prominence in the plaque implicates neuronal degeneration as playing an important role in the pathogenesis of the plaque.

The fibril-filled dendrites and axons correspond to the strongly argentophilic fibers seen in classical silver preparations. These neuronal processes have been affected by an overproduction of neurofilaments, just as have some neuronal perikarya. The closely packed, well-oriented neurofilaments contribute to the birefringence of the plaque as do the amyloid bundles.

Schmitt [25] proposed, on the basis of a series of biophysical and biochemical experiments, that a neurofibril is made up of a group of protofilaments. He believed that the latter are each a chain of 30 Å globular proteins, and that these chains are twisted in a slow helix around an empty core to form the 100 Å wide neurofilament. The electron microscopic image of filaments in our material corresponds very closely to the hypothetical model presented by Schmitt and by Davison and Taylor.[30]

Kidd [26] has more recently suggested that the triple contour of the neurofibril is due to its being made up of a pair of closely parallel, regularly twisted protofibrils. The longitudinal sections of neurofilaments could not dispute this concept, but cross sections do not reveal paired structures. There are, rather, circlets and triple density curved elements. The latter might indicate curvature of the filament in the thickness of the section.

The birefringence of the neurofibrillary tangle is undoubtedly related to the excellent orientation of the filaments within the clusters. The congophilia of the same structure is less easily explicable, for the tangle, as we have seen it, is clearly not composed of amyloid. Nevertheless, the component neurofibrils are of a width very similar to that of amyloid fibrils. Ghidoni and Gueft [19] have suggested that staining by Congo red might be based on some relationship between this diameter and the size of the dye molecules. That the dye molecules are physically arranged in an ordered fashion in the filaments is shown by the increased birefringence of a tangle stained with Congo red.

The ultrastructural aspects of wallerian degeneration in the peripheral nervous system are well known.[12,13] Similar phenomena have been found [14] in the cerebrum in Tay-Sachs disease, where secondary demyelinization is to be expected. The characteristics of primary myelin degeneration in the central nervous system have not, however, been described. Furthermore, primary demyelinization is not generally recognized in Alzheimer's disease.

Nonetheless, our micrographs clearly show intact axons surrounded by bubbled and granular myelin sheaths. They seem to indicate myelin disruption without axonal disorder and this, by definition, is primary demyelinization. The additional presence of digestion chambers with degenerative axoplasm might indicate either a later stage of the same process or a concomitant wallerian degeneration. The latter would presumably be secondary to neuronal death. These processes could account for the frequently noticed but rarely discussed shrinkage of cerebral white matter in senile and presenile dementia.

The vascular changes presented a striking picture which is without adequate precedent. Majno and Palade [27] showed gaps arising between venular endothelial cells in muscle when serotonin was injected locally. Casley-Smith [28] showed similar gaps between the lining cells of jejunal lacteals in animals fed quantities of lipid. Furthermore, vesicles, identified by isolation studies as representing chylomicrons, were found within these latter gaps. He considered these vesicles to be moving into the lumen of the lymphatics. The chylomicrons were of an appearance identical to the vesicles found in venular endothelial fenestrae in our material. Casley-Smith also described smaller dense particles, identified as lipoprotein, in caveolae on the luminal surface of the lacteal lining cells. These were invaginations into the cytoplasm, rather than, as in the tissue we have described, evaginations from cytoplasm into lumen. These granule-filled evaginations are apparently unique, and previous reference to them has not been found. Movat and Fernando [29] described dense precipitates within the lumens of sensitized mesenteric vessels one minute after exposure to antigen. However, the precipitates were unbounded, were not connected with the endothelium and were seen to move through endothelial gaps from lumen to adjacent tissue.

The central nervous system, as is well known, lacks lymphatics. Nevertheless, because of its large component of structural lipids, the brain might be called upon to transport quantities of fats in instances, for example, of destructive disease. Although catabolic cellular activity undoubtedly accounts for most lipid breakdown, it is not impossible that some large molecules would be carried to vessels by ameboid cells and then pass in aggregates through the wall to enter the lumen. It is suggested that the vesicles within the interendothelial gaps in the cere-

226

bral cortex in Alzheimer's disease might represent chylomicron-containing, alcohol-soluble, neutral lipids, bound in a phospholipid membrane, and that lipoproteins might make up the granules in the endothelial excrescences and intraluminal deposits. Both lipids might be catabolic products of degenerating myelin and neurons caught in the process of transport across vascular walls. These mechanisms are not to be considered specific for Alzheimer's disease, and it is expected that the vascular changes will be found in other situations in the brain and probably in other organs as well.

Summary

Cerebral biopsy specimens from 3 patients with Alzheimer's presenile dementia were examined by electron microscopy. Four major morphologic features were studied in detail: senile plaque, neurofibrillary tangle, myelin degeneration and endothelial modification.

The plaques had a core of amyloid fibrils. Large dendrites and axons with an excess of neurofilaments surrounded the core. Also prominent were neuronal processes which contained many laminated dense bodies. Microglia were present and seemed to be the source of the amyloid.

Alzheimer's neurofibrillary tangles were made up of great numbers of closely packed, normal neurofilaments which displaced the other cytoplasmic organelles within affected neuronal perikarya.

Myelin degeneration was often found without axonal degeneration. Wallerian degeneration was also noted.

Certain small vessels displayed endothelial fenestrations in which were several chylomicron-like vesicles. Dense particulate aggregates, possibly lipoprotein in nature, were seen to protrude from the endothelium into the lumen.

Addendum

It has been very recently learned by the authors that the third patient had familial hyperlipemia, with elevation of serum cholesterol, phospholipid and total lipid. The altered vessels were found only in the tissue from this patient. It is our opinion that the endothelial changes described here are related to the familial hyperlipemia rather than the Alzheimer's disease.

References

1. TERRY, R. D., and WEISS, M. Studies in Tay-Sachs disease. A. Methods. 2. Electron microscopic. *J. Neuropath. & Exper. Neurol.*, 1963, 22, 2–9.
2. GOMORI, G. Microscopic Histochemistry: Principles and Practice. Univ. of Chicago Press, Chicago, 1952.

3. NOVIKOFF, A. B. Lysosomes and the physiology and pathology of cells. (Abstract) *Biol. Bull.*, 1959, 117, 385.

4. NOVIKOFF, A. B., and GOLDFISCHER, S. Nucleosidediphosphatase activity in the Golgi apparatus and its usefulness for cytologic studies. *Proc. Nat. Acad. Sc.*, 1961, 47, 802–810.

5. PALADE, G. E. A study of fixation for electron microscopy. *J. Exper. Med.*, 1952, 95, 285–298.

6. CAULFIELD, J. B. Effects of varying the vehicle for OsO$_4$ in tissue fixation. *J. Biophys. & Biochem. Cytol.*, 1957, 3, 827–830.

7. LUFT, J. H. Improvements in epoxy resin embedding methods. *J. Biophys. & Biochem. Cytol.*, 1961, 9, 409–414.

8. WEBSTER, H. D.; SPIRO, D.; WAKSMAN, B., and ADAMS, R. D. Phase and electron microscopic studies of experimental demyelination. II. Schwann cell changes in guinea pig sciatic nerves during experimental diphtheritic neuritis. *J. Neuropath. & Exper. Neurol.*, 1961, 20, 5–34.

9. MILLONIG, G. A modified procedure for lead staining of thin sections. *J. Biophys. & Biochem. Cytol.*, 1961, 11, 736–739.

10. HUXLEY, H. E., and ZUBAY, G. Preferential staining of nucleic acid-containing structures for electron miscoscopy. *J. Biophys. & Biochem. Cytol.*, 1961, 11, 273–296.

11. TERRY, R. D. The fine structure of neurofibrillary tangles in Alzheimer's disease. *J. Neuropath. & Exper. Neurol.*, 1963, 22, 629–642.

12. VIAL, J. D. The early changes in the axoplasm during wallerian degeneration. *J. Biophys. & Biochem. Cytol.*, 1958, 4, 551–555.

13. TERRY, R. D., and HARKIN, J. C. Wallerian Degeneration and Regeneration of Peripheral Nerves. In: The Biology of Myelin. KOREY, S. R. (ed.) Paul B. Hoeber, Inc., New York, 1959, pp. 303–320.

14. TERRY, R. D., and WEISS, M. Studies in Tay-Sachs disease. II. Ultrastructure of the cerebrum. *J. Neuropath. & Exper. Neurol.*, 1963, 22, 18–55.

15. MARGOLIS, G. Senile cerebral disease. A critical survey of traditional concepts based upon observations with newer technics. *Lab. Invest.*, 1959, 8, 335–370.

16. DIVRY, P. De la nature de l'altération fibrillaire d'Alzheimer. *J. belge de neurol. et psychiat.*, 1934, 34, 197–201.

17. DIVRY, P., and FLORKIN, M. Sur les propriétés optiques d l'amyloïde. *Compt. rend. Soc. biol.*, 1927, 97, 1808–1810.

18. COHEN, A. S.; WEISS, L., and CALKINS, E. Electron microscopic observations of the spleen during the induction of experimental amyloidosis in the rabbit. *Am. J. Path.*, 1960, 37, 413–431.

19. GHIDONI, J., and GUEFT, B. The Double Nature of the Amyloid Fiber. In: Electron Microscopy. Fifth International Congress for Electron Microscopy, 1962. BREESE, S. S., JR. (ed.). Academic Press, Inc., New York, 1962, Vol. 2, T-15.

20. HEEFNER, W. A., and SORENSON, G. D. Experimental amyloidosis. I. Light and electron microscopic observations of spleen and lymph nodes. *Lab. Invest.*, 1962, 11, 585–593.

21. TRUMP, B. F., and BENDITT, E. P. Electron microscopic studies of human renal disease. Observations of normal visceral glomerular epithelium and its modification in disease. *Lab. Invest.*, 1962, 11, 753–781.

22. GONATAS, N. K.; KOREY, S. R.; TERRY, R. D.; GOMEZ, C.; WINKLER, R., and STEIN, A. A case of juvenile lipidosis—electron microscopic and biochemical

observations of a cerebral biopsy and their significance. *J. Neuropath. & Exper. Neurol.*, 1963, 22, 557–580.

23. TERRY, R. D., and GONATAS, N. K.   Unpublished data.
24. WEBSTER, H. D.   Transient, focal accumulation of axonal mitochondria during the early stages of wallerian degeneration. *J. Cell Biol.*, 1962, 12, 361–383.
25. SCHMITT, F. O.   Biologie moléculaire des neurofilaments. In: Actualités Neuro-physiologiques. MONNIER, A. (ed.). Masson & Cie, Paris, 1962.
26. KIDD, M.   Paired helical filaments in electron microscopy of Alzheimer's disease. *Nature, London*, 1963, 197, 192–193.
27. MAJNO, G., and PALADE, G. E.   Studies on inflammation. I. The effect of histamine and serotonin on vascular permeability; an electron microscope study. *J. Biophys. & Biochem. Cytol.*, 1961, 11, 571–605.
28. CASLEY-SMITH, J. R.   The identification of chylomicra and lipoproteins in tissue sections and their passage into jejunal lacteals. *J. Cell Biol.*, 1962, 15, 259–277.
29. MOVAT, H. Z., and FERNANDO, N. V. P.   Allergic inflammation. I. The earliest fine structural changes at the blood-tissue barrier during antigen-antibody interaction. *Am. J. Path.*, 1963, 42, 41–59.
30. DAVISON, P. F., and TAYLOR, E. W.   Physical-chemical studies of proteins of squid nerve axoplasm, with special reference to the axon fibrous protein. *J. Gen. Physiol.*, 1960, 43, 801–823.

The authors are grateful to the members of the Departments of Neurology and Neurosurgery who cared for the patients, for providing the biopsy specimens.

We wish to thank Dr. S. R. Korey for his stimulus and advice, Dr. A. A. Angrist for his editorial assistance, and Mrs. Robyn Shoulson and Mrs. Norma Marmor for their technical assistance.

[*Illustrations follow*]

229

LEGENDS FOR FIGURES

Key:

AF = astrocyte foot process	L = lipid
AM = amyloid fibrils	LF = lipofuscin
AP = fibrous process of astrocyte	LU = lumen
AX = axoplasm	M = mitochondrion
BM = basement membrane	N = nucleus
C = chylomicron-like vesicle	NF = neurofibrils
DB = dense bodies	NP = neuronal process
ES = extracellular space	P = perithelial cell
G = Golgi apparatus	R = ribosomes
GF = glial fibrils	RBC = red blood cell

Fig. 1.   A senile plaque shows a central core of amyloid, large neuronal processes, dense bodies and a single cell. × 4,400.

Fig. 2.   A senile plaque exhibits similar elements. The cell contains numerous lipid bodies. × 5,500.

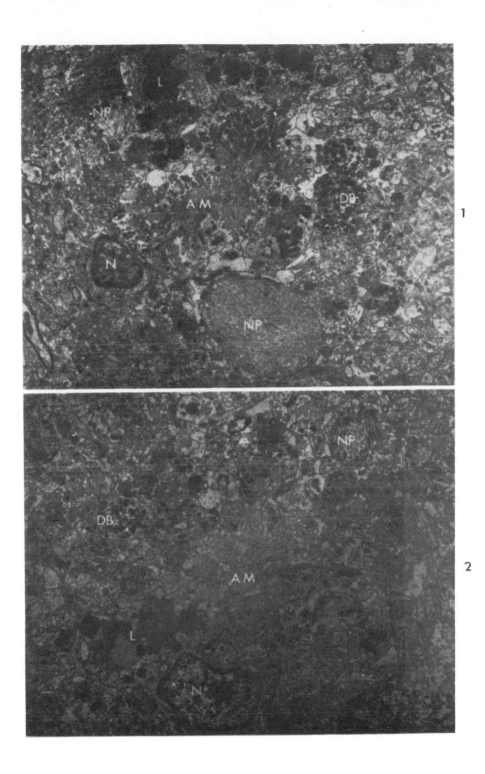

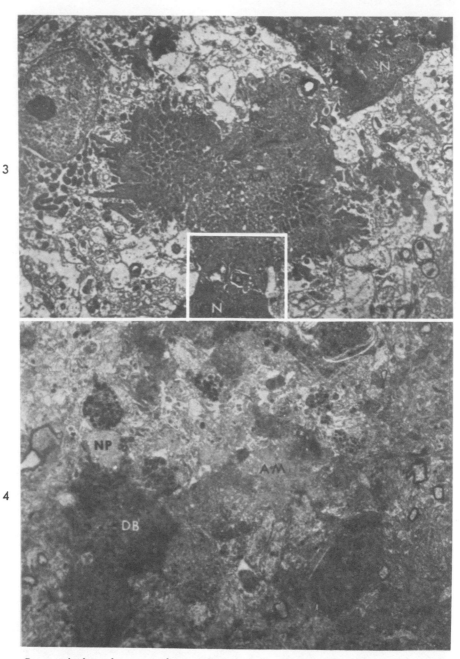

FIG. 3. A plaque has a very dense, stellate amyloid core. This material is related to the cells at left and at bottom. × 5,100.

FIG. 4. Another plaque exhibits especially prominent aggregates of dense bodies. × 4,900.

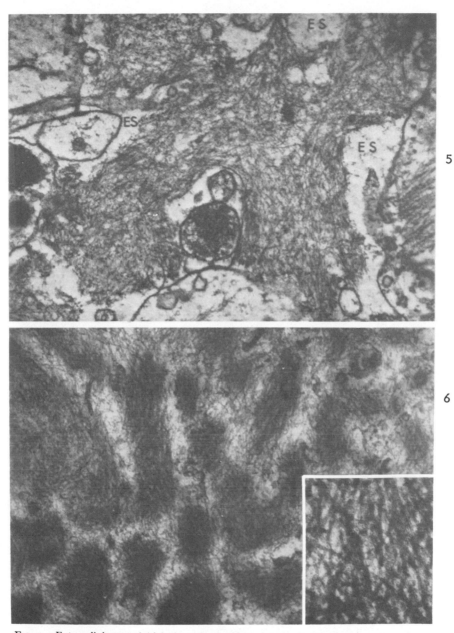

FIG. 5. Extracellular amyloid lacks a boundary membrane in apposition to the several circumscribed cell processes. × 39,000.

FIG. 6. A portion of the amyloid core from Figure 5. In the bundles are interwoven but oriented fibers. × 51,000. The inset demonstrates the hollow structure of the amyloid filaments. × 120,000.

233

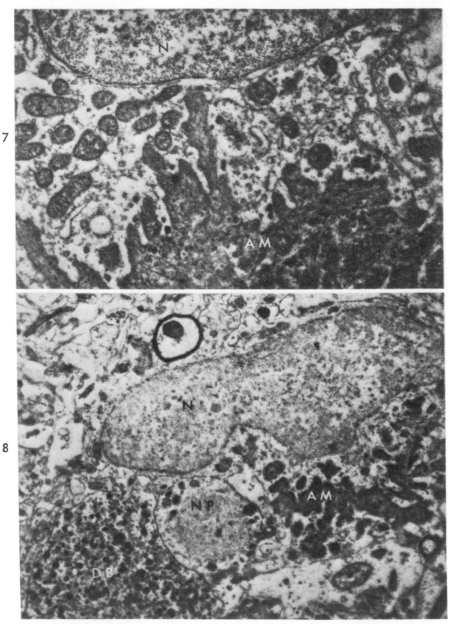

FIG. 7.   A detail from the left of Figure 3. The amyloid bundles lie in deep indentations of the cell and are partially separated from the cytoplasm by an incomplete membrane. X 19,000.

FIG. 8.   This cell has many unbounded amyloid bundles in its cytoplasm. A neuronal process with many neurofibrils and a large aggregate of dense bodies lie nearby. X 11,000.

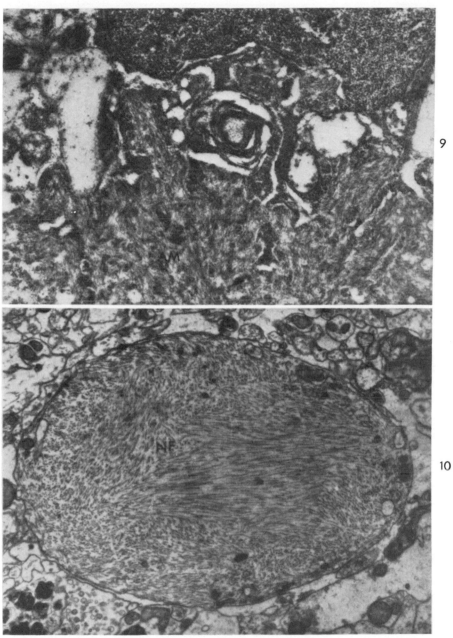

9

10

FIG. 9.   A detail from bottom of Figure 3. The basophilic cytoplasm extends in tongues among the masses of amyloid. × 25,000.

FIG. 10.   A distended neuronal process is filled with neurofibrils. This is a detail from Figure 1. × 12,000.

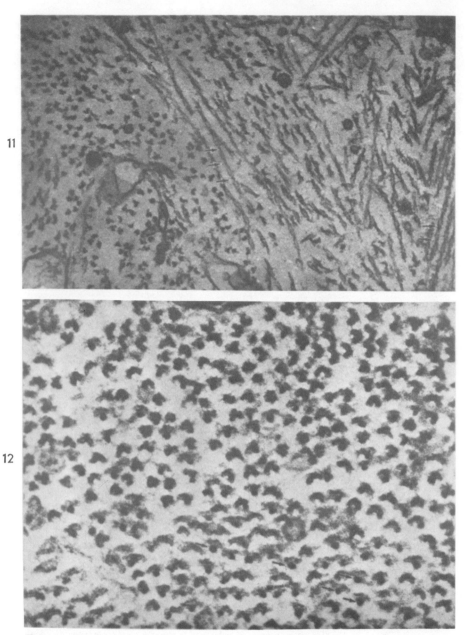

FIG. 11. Numbers of neurofilaments appear in longitudinal sections at the right, and in cross section at the left. The former show intermittent narrowing (arrows) which might indicate twists. × 57,000.

FIG. 12. Neurofilaments cut in cross section. Most have curved, triple density outline, but some (arrows) have circular profiles. × 140,000.

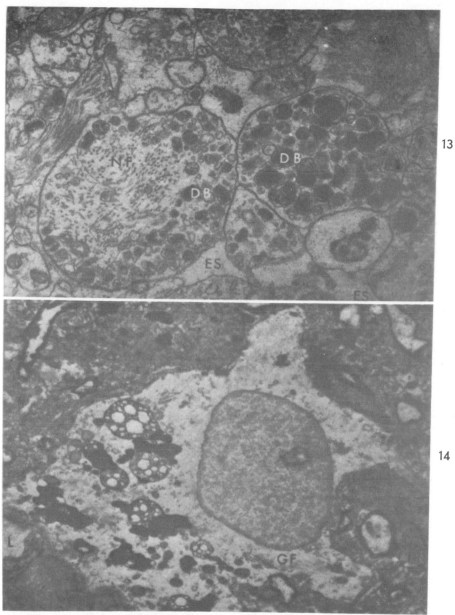

13

14

FIG. 13. The cell process on the left contains neurofilaments and peripheral dense bodies. Immediately to the right is a cell process filled with partially laminated dense bodies. Extracellular amyloid is present at top right. Extracellular space is apparent. × 22,000.

FIG. 14. This enlarged astrocyte is adjacent to a vessel (lower left) and contains bundles of glial fibrils and several vesiculated lipid bodies. The neuropil is compact. × 9,300.

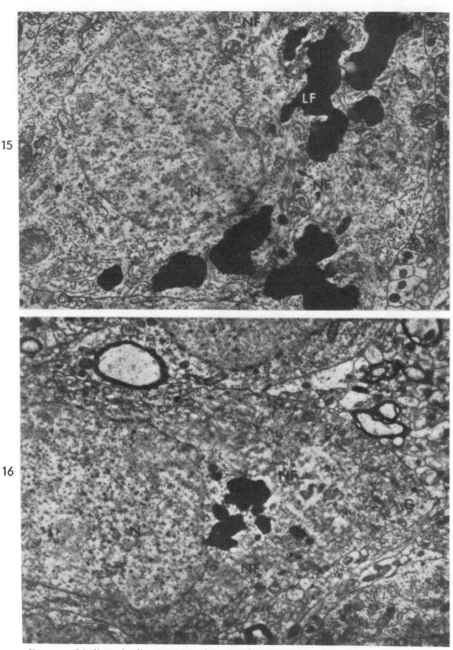

FIG. 15. Medium-sized neuron contains a moderate number of lipofuscin bodies. Neurofibrillary aggregates are mildly increased above normal. × 11,000.

FIG. 16. A neuron displays a moderately severe tangle of neurofibrils. × 9,600.

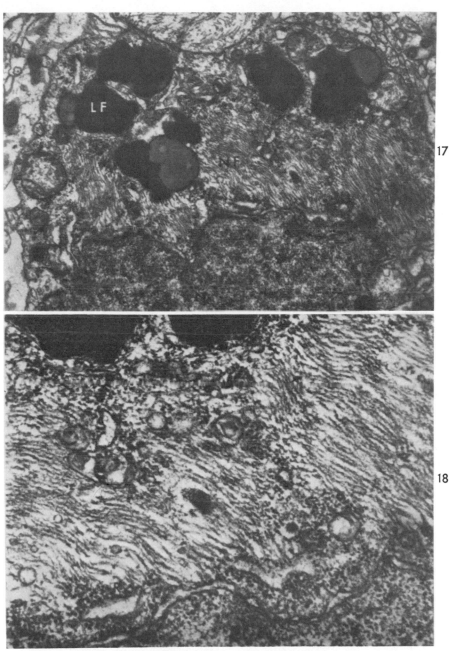

FIG. 17. Most of the cytoplasm of this smaller neuron has been displaced by the extensive neurofibrillary tangle. × 18,000.

FIG. 18. Higher magnification of Figure 17. × 47,000.

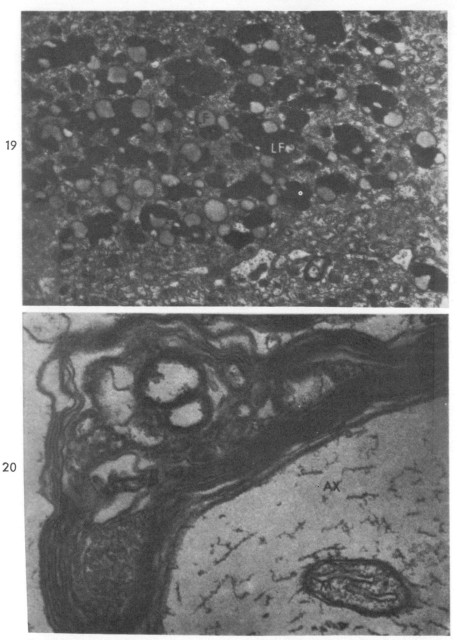

FIG. 19. A neuron contains a great many lipofuscin bodies, but its neurofibrillary content is not remarkable. × 9,000.

FIG. 20. Abnormal myelin with lamellar and granular degeneration surrounds a normal axon. × 76,000.

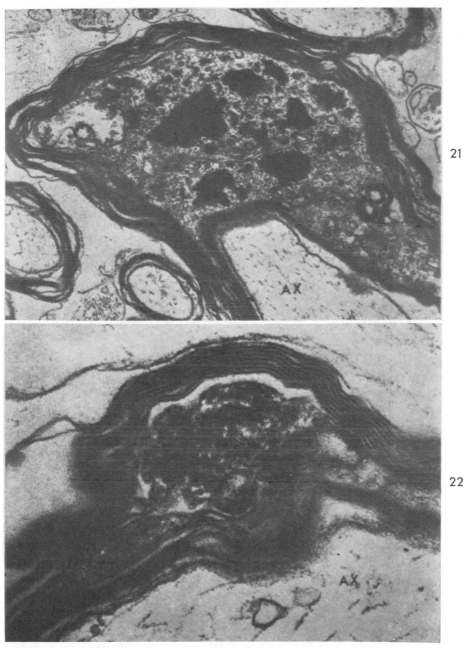

FIG. 21. Severe but focal granular degeneration of myelin is associated with an intact axis cylinder. × 27,000.

FIG. 22. Granular myelin degeneration in the presence of a normal axon. × 86,000.

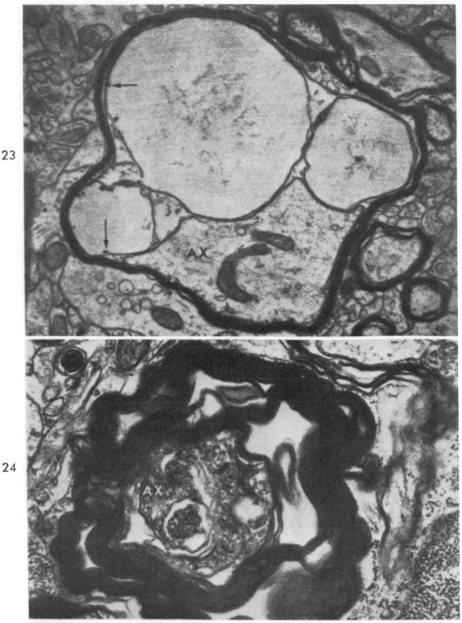

FIG. 23.   This myelin sheath is normal. Several large vacuoles compress the otherwise unremarkable axis cylinder. The abnormal vacuoles are bounded by membranes which are occasionally broken and knotted (arrows). × 25,000.

FIG. 24.   A later stage of axonal degeneration. The axoplasm is dense and granular; the myelin is broken and crumpled although still laminated. × 33,000.

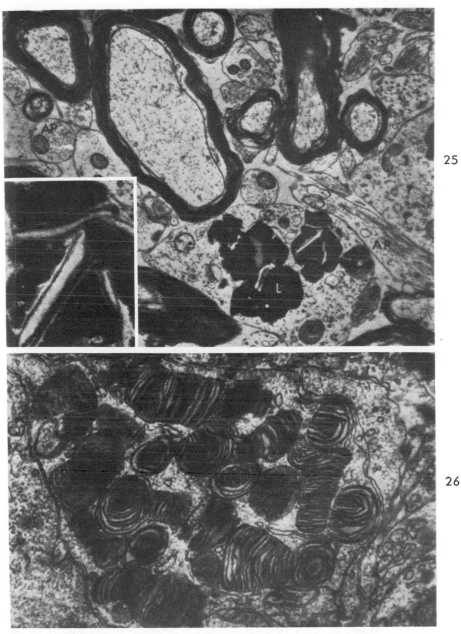

FIG. 25. Glial processes in the white matter occasionally contain dense lipid. × 16,000. The inset reveals its partially lamellated structure. × 60,000.

FIG. 26. Occasional aggregates of lamellar lipid bodies are found. These closely resemble the membranous cytoplasmic bodies of Tay-Sachs disease. × 34,000.

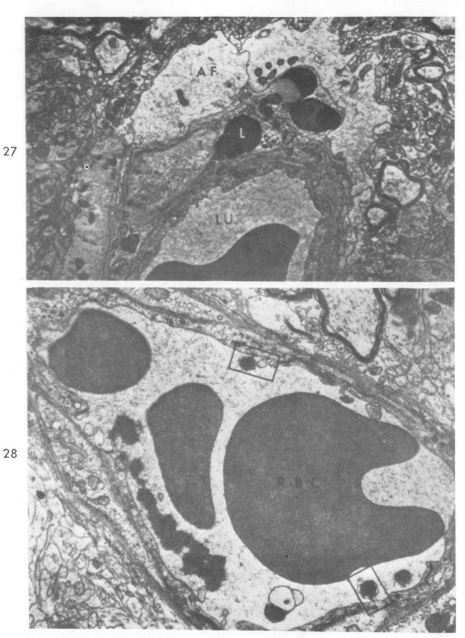

FIG. 27. Several astrocytic foot processes closely surround the upper aspect of this vessel. A perithelial cell contains several lipid droplets. × 9,700.

FIG. 28. A small vessel contains numerous dense, unbounded aggregates in its lumen. The endothelium displays an excrescence at the bottom and a membrane-gap at the top. Each contains dense particulate material similar to that in the lumen. × 13,000.

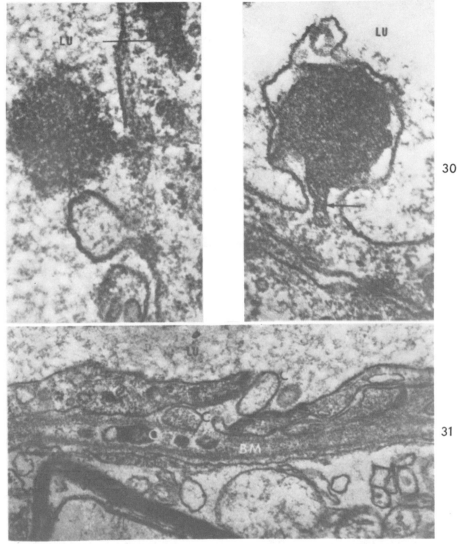

29

30

31

FIG. 29. Detail from top of Figure 28. The lumen is to the left, the endothelium at the
right. The lumen membrane is invaginated into the lumen at the bottom and is broken
in the middle. Dense material appears in the endothelial cytoplasm (arrow) and pro-
trudes from the endothelium into the lumen through the break. × 95,000.

FIG. 30. Detail from bottom of Figure 28. The endothelial excrescence extends upward
into the lumen. It is bounded by the lumen membrane. Dense material fills the evagina-
tion and is itself partly surrounded by a unit membrane (arrow). × 95,000.

FIG. 31. The endothelial cells lining this vessel are separated by a gap in which are
several vesicles resembling chylomicrons. These seem to extend from the basement
membrane into the lumen. × 43,000.

245

Alzheimer's Disease

W. Hughes

With the increase in the proportion of elderly people in the community we must expect an increase in the incidence of those diseases which occur more frequently in the higher age groups. One of the most important of these, by reason of its high and increasing prevalence, is that originally described as a rare form of pre-senile dementia by ALZHEIMER in 1907. There has been a good deal of confusion about the name and identity of this disease. The case Alzheimer described was in a woman aged 51 who developed a progressive dementia and died after 5 years. The significant histological feature in the brain was the presence of large numbers of argyrophilic plaques and neurofibrillary degenerative changes (NFD) which were found throughout the cerebral cortex.

The typical argyrophilic plaque is a large lesion which may be just visible to the naked eye in stained sections. In well prepared sections typical plaques and NFD are easy to recognise. There are also present in most cases many amorphous argyrophilic particles – 'Alzheimer material' – which cannot be identified with individual plaques or NFD but which might derive from either source. For a while it was believed that NFD was a specific lesion and in the literature it is often called the Alzheimer degeneration.

In 1910 FISCHER published his account of presbyophrenic dementia. In 275 necropsies on elderly subjects with mental disease he found Alzheimer changes in 58 cases. The symptoms and lesions in the latter corresponded fairly well with those in the case described by ALZHEIMER. Plaques were found in every instance and NFD in 19 cases. The majority of his cases were over 75; in fact one of them was 103 years old.

Even if we allow a duration of 10 years before death there could be no question of labelling this disease pre-senile dementia. Right from the beginning the relationship between Fischer's presbyophrenia, old age and Alzheimer's disease has been the subject of controversy.

REDLICH [1898] has a special claim to priority in the identification of the disease. He found plaques in a case which he described as one of senile dementia. The patient who was 78 years old at the time of her death had epileptiform fits during the last year of her life and for this reason the case is usually referred to as one of senile epilepsy in the literature. Apart from the fits the case had all the significant clinical features of the disease later described by ALZHEIMER.

GRUNTHAL [1933] examined the brains of 13 patients diagnosed as Alzheimer's disease by various clinicians and in every one he found the typical plaques and NFD. He also found a good correlation between clinical and pathological findings. The concentration of plaques and NFD paralleled the severity of symptoms during life. This suggested that Alzheimer's disease was a well defined entity which could be identified by careful clinical examination and confirmed by pathological findings and particularly by the finding of large numbers of plaques and NFD in the cortex.

Aging and Alzheimer's Disease

An important contribution came from GELLERSTEDT [1933] who examined the brains of 50 'normal' old people. He took the greatest care to exclude any neurological or psychological taint in the symptoms during life or in the cause of death. All died from the common causes of death in old age – cancer, myocardial degeneration, chronic bronchitis, acute or chronic sepsis. To make the study more exact he studied the brains of 50 'controls' – children, adolescents and elderly psychotics. The chief result of this painstaking study was the finding of plaques and NFD in the brains of over 80% of 'normal' old people. In some cases the concentration was as high as those reported by previous observers in Alzheimer's disease. GELLERSTEDT's findings suggested that the presence of plaques and NFD even in high concentration could not define the boundaries between Alzheimer's disease and the changes which occur in the aged brain. Some of the discrepancies here are semantic in origin and hinge on the difficulty of identifying and defining the norm in old age.

SIMCHOVITZ [1911, 1914] had already suggested counting the plaques and this procedure has been advocated by subsequent observers to establish the diagnosis of Alzheimer's disease. While it is true that in general the concentration of plaques parallels the severity of the disease, the correlation is by no means exact. In some advanced cases of the disease plaques and NFD may be quite scarce.

In spite of the apparent discrepancy in the matter of age most authors [NEWTON, 1948; ROTHSCHILD, 1937; McMENEMEY, 1963] now regard Alzheimer's pre-senile dementia and Fischer's presbyophrenic dementia as variants of the same disease. Unfortunately up to the present it has been impossible to agree on a name for the condition. In the literature generally authors use the term dementia to cover forms of mental deterioration associated with identifiable neurological lesions and psychosis for mental disease in which no organic lesions has yet been identified. According to this convention Alzheimer's disease is a form of pre-senile or senile dementia. Throughout the literature however senile psychosis is the term which is more frequently used for the presbyophrenic form described by FISCHER. This goes against the convention and in any case it is not a good name for the Alzheimer variant which occurs in younger subjects. It should be mentioned however that some authors call the Fischer variant senile dementia. FISCHER himself wanted to call the disease *Sphaerocytosis cerebri multiplex* but the name did not stick.

The lack of an agreed name is holding up the recognition of the disease at clinical level. The incidence reported by pathologists from *post mortem* data in mental hospitals ranges from 1.2% [McMENEMEY, 1963] to 27% [WOODARD, 1966]. The Registrar General's statistics are quite misleading since they only show a total of 135 deaths in England and Wales in 1964 under Section 305 of the International List of Causes of Death. This section includes Alzheimer's and Pick's disease and other forms of cerebral atrophy. Since we find that most of the patients are labelled cerebral arteriosclerosis during life the cause of death is probably classified under the heading of vascular diseases of the brain in Sections 330–4. In the most popular English textbook of medicine there is no mention of the name of Alzheimer nor Fischer. Presbyophrenia is not mentioned nor is there any attempt to differentiate senile psychosis clinically from the mass of organic senile dementia. An additional reason for the low figure from the Registrar General is the fact that Alzheimer patients usually die from intercurrent disease.

248

From the foregoing it will be understood that the disease as we see it among the elderly population is Redlich's or Fischer's rather than Alzheimer's disease. Nevertheless many aspects of the disease continue to be overshadowed by the name of Alzheimer; there is the Alzheimer change in cells, NFD is the Alzheimer lesion, the basic substance of the plaques is Alzheimer material, the pathological process Alzheimerisation. We have thought it better to retain the title of Alzheimer's disease for the condition we wish to describe in this paper.

An original observation which may go a long way to solve this problem was made by Divry in 1927 when he reported that the ground substance of the plaque had all the histochemical characteristics of amyloid including bi-refringence with appropriate staining. This observation which did not attract much attention at the time has acquired a new significance in view of the current conception of the nature of amyloid and its relation to immunity on the one hand and aging on the other.

Material

The following account is based mainly on a clinical study of 96 cases observed in this hospital over the past 10 years. Although the first case was observed in 1959, I was hesitant about arriving at a diagnosis of Alzheimer's disease in similar cases especially when the patient was over the age of 75 years. When the clinical diagnosis was confirmed repeatedly by pathological findings *post mortem* it was obvious that we were dealing with a very common disease which could be diagnosed with a high degree of certainty during life. Nevertheless there must always be some doubt about a diagnosis which is not confirmed by positive neuropathological findings *post mortem*. Our series of cases can be split into diagnostic categories of varying probability.

Group A. This is a definitive group of 14 females and 5 males cases (table I) all of whom were confirmed by macroscopic and histological investigation of the brain *post mortem*. A small group of 3 females and 2 males in this Group showed plaques and neurofibrillary changes on biopsy and one of these female cases was further confirmed at *post mortem*.

Cerebral atrophy is an important diagnostic feature which can be demonstrated by an air encephalogram during life. Most of our cases were unsuitable for one reason or another for such investigation. *Post mortem*, cerebral atrophy is confirmed particularly by loss of brain weight and dilatation of the ventricles.

Table I

	Total	Age of onset (years) Mean	(Range)	Brain weight (grams) Mean	(Range)
Female	14	74	(65–85)	1,025	(840–1,334)
Male	5	63	(55–78)	1,125	(1,070–1,190)

Table II

	Total	Age of onset		Brain weight	
		Mean	(Range)	Mean	(Range)
Female	21	73	(64–96)	1,050	(950–1,300)
Male	9	70	(57–87)	1,208	(1,070–1,360)

Table III

	Total	Age of onset	
		Mean	(Range)
Female	37	79	(62–89)
Male	10	72	(58–82)

Group B comprises 21 females and 9 males all cases in which clinical findings during life are supplemented by finding some degree of cerebral atrophy *post mortem* as shown in table II.

Group C contains 47 cases, 37 females and 10 males – diagnosed on clinical and laboratory findings only. In all cases these will include negative serological tests for syphilis and abnormal electro-encephalographic (EEG) tracing.

Prevalence

For many reasons it is difficult to assess the prevalence of the disease in the community. Owing to its chronicity and the nature of the symptoms typical cases tend to accumulate in hospital and the disease is a major cause of bed occupancy on our geriatric wards. At the time of writing there were in my own wards 19 cases (1 confirmed by cortical biopsy) among 99 females patients and 3 cases (1 confirmed by cortical biopsy) among 35 males. These are not included in the groups above. If we round off these figures to 20% of females and 8% of males this would, I think, give a fair estimate of the prevalence of the disease in geriatric hospital wards. This of course does not take into account the beds occupied in mental hospitals by Alzheimer patients. The reported incidence in females is always higher than in males and this is borne out by our own figures.

Onset and Duration

The onset of the disease is difficult to determine since we must depend on the observations of relatives and these are notoriously inaccurate and often contradictory. Subject to this qualification the figures above show the age of onset in the three diagnostic categories. In the whole series of 96 cases the age of onset in 6 of the 72 females and in 4 of the 24 males was below 65 years.

The duration as observed in hospital varies widely. One case still living has been in hospital for over 8 years. The minimum total duration of the disease as far as our observations go is not less than 1 year. The mean duration for the combined Groups A and B is just over 3 years.

We found no correlation between age of onset and brain weight nor, surprisingly between duration of disease and brain weight in the microscopically confirmed cases.

Clinical Features

To illustrate the main clinical features 2 cases are given in some detail below. The first is an Alzheimer type with onset before the age of 65 and the other a Fischer type which started after the age of 70 years.

Case 1

Widowed school mistress aged 65. Seen in her own home 16.12.1963. She had two children, one unmarried daughter with whom she lived and a married son, both healthy.

History of forgetfulness going back certainly for 2 years, possibly much longer. Had been living alone but became quite incapable of looking after herself and her daughter had to give up work to come and live with her. She was ambulant and if left alone would go out and get lost. Several times neighbours or the police had brought her home. She made frequent mistakes in dressing and had become careless in her habits. In the lavatory she had often used a handkerchief or table napkin after defaecation putting this with the rest of the clothes for the wash.

On admission to hospital, 19.12.1963, she was ambulant and needed only a little help in dressing and in feeding. Left to herself she would eat with her fingers. She was restless day and night and tended to wander if not watched.

Physically she was well nourished and examination of respiratory cardiovascular and alimentary systems revealed no abnormality. Neurologically her tendon and plantar reflexes were normal and sensation appeared to be normal. A 'snout' reflex – pouting of the lips when the skin was flicked with a finger – and occasionally a sucking reflex could be elicited. There were no ocular changes. The memory defect was severe. She could not remember the name of the hospital nor her address before admission. She never learned which was her own bed in the ward nor where the lavatory was. She remembered only a few words of French although she had taught the language in school at one time. She smiled when spoken to but did not initiate any conversation. She confabulated freely. Her answers to questions were stereotyped.

Laboratory findings: Blood – red and white cell counts within normal limits; urea 26 mg per 100 ml; total serum proteins 6.3 g, albumin 2.59, globulin 3.8 g per 100 ml. Electrophoresis showed an increase in the a-2 globulins. Serological tests for syphilis negative; latex globulin spot test negative; no LE cells.

EEG. Record outside normal limits displaying general excess of slow activity; a rhythm absent frontal and parietal regions.

Cortical biopsy – 25.8.1966. A piece of cortex from the parietal lobe was sectioned and revealed plaques and NFD typical of Alzheimer's disease.

In hospital her condition slowly deteriorated; after one year her speech had become jargon with a peculiar fragmentation of sentences. Her appetite diminished and she began to lose weight. She became spastic and bedfast, developed contractures and finally pressure sores. She died 13 months after the cortical biopsy and 2 years 4 months after admission to hospital.

Post mortem – the significant findings were: (1) Cerebral atrophy; the brain weighed 950 g; (2) pulmonary embolism from thrombosis of leg veins which was the immediate cause of death; (3) almost complete absence of arteriosclerotic lesions in the systemic and cerebral vessels.

Case 2

Housewife aged 78 admitted to Manor Park Hospital on 31.5.1966 with a history of recent stroke attributed to cerebral arteriosclerosis. The patient had been found unconscious in bed one morning a week before admission. She recovered consciousness the same afternoon and there was no residual paralysis. Her elderly husband had observed behavioural changes going back over 5 years. She had become increasingly forgetful, aggressive, confused and restless. She had wandered outside and got lost many times.

On admission she was amnesic, ambulant and restless. The amnesia had all the usual characteristics. She resisted examination and particularly resented questions – 'Why do you keep on at me?' Physical examination and X-ray chest revealed no abnormalities in cardiovascular, respiratory or digestive systems. Blood pressure 120/80 mmHg. Her tendon reflexes were normal and there were no ocular changes. The plantar reflexes were flexor. A 'snout' reflex could be elicited.

Laboratory investigations: Blood – haemoglobin 14.8 g urea 40 mg, total serum proteins 6.8 g, globulin 3.1 g, albumin 3.7 g per 100 ml; white cells 7,300 with normal distribution; Wasserman reaction negative. Urine – no abnormalities.

EEG. An abnormal record displaying a generalised excess of slow activity. The pattern suggested diffuse organic change.

She remained fully ambulant and tended to wander from the ward. She was given up to 300 mg chlorpromazine daily. She developed jaundice on this dosage but it cleared up as soon as the drug was replaced by promazine. Cortical biopsy revealed typical histological changes of Alzheimer's disease including plaques and NFD. Electronmicroscopy confirmed the presence of amyloid neurofibrillary changes.

Her mental and physical condition seemed to improve for a while after the biopsy but on 5.4.1967 she developed herpes zoster in the lumbar region and began to deteriorate. She became spastic – a grasp reflex and sucking reflex could be elicited and she began rubbing and tapping. The tapping with her fingers went on day after day and necessitated heavy sedation to keep her quiet. She developed a speech defect characterised chiefly by inability to complete a sentence. She gradually lost weight and became very emaciated before death. She developed influenza at the peak of the 1967/1968 winter epidemic and died on 14.1.1968. At *post mortem* the brain weight was 1,150 g.

The onset, development and final clinical picture are much the same in the two cases. The difference in age at onset puts one in the pre-senile and the other in the senile group but we are obviously dealing with the same disease in both cases. The main symptoms – amnesia, motor restlessness and dysphasia are commonplace enough and characterise many forms of disease in old age. Nevertheless a careful appraisal of what we have actually observed reveals semeiological characteristics which are highly specific and which, alone or in combination, can lead to a firm diagnosis during life in most cases.

Amnesia dominates the clinical picture particularly in the early stage. The onset is gradual and it may be very difficult to identify the point of disease in elderly subjects who are universally forgetful. It is difficult to describe amnesia without getting bogged down among the ambiguous terms and ill-defined concepts which abound in this field. It is a complex psychological state in which we see the basic defect as inability to learn. The patient cannot retain fresh information although like the Korsakovian amnesic she can still utilise it. In the early years of the disease the patient can play a game of draughts or chess or provide rational arguments in a discussion and distinguish right from wrong [LHERMITTE, 1924]. Confabulation in this stage is a conscious attempt to cover up the memory defect. The patient tries to go along with the examiner as far as possible. It is the ability to do this which gives the amnesia a characteristic twist. Skills and knowledge acquired in youth or in the distant past are retained to some extent until late in the disease. Hence the patient can integrate information to an extent which often deceives relatives and goes a long way to conceal the basic amnesic defect. A simple but very efficient test which we often employ brings out this point. The patient is given a four digit number to remember as the hospital telephone number. She is asked to repeat the telephone number after about 15 sec. At this stage she cannot recall the number but will point out that there is no necessity to do so since the number is in the telephone directory. While integrative function is largely intact in the early stages the ability to remember and recall is lacking.

In younger subjects still at work the inability to remember will soon lead to loss of employment. In elderly subjects in which the early symptoms occur in the years after retirement it will begin to show in forgetfulness leading to deterioration in personal habits, carelessness in dressing, lack of cleanliness in the home. There are arguments about money or personal property which is lost, mislaid or forgotten. There are recurrent quarrels with shopkeepers about the correct change after purchases. The patient lights the gas and forgets to turn it off. For obvious reasons this can be dangerous with a coin-operated meter. A daughter at this stage will often bring the patient to live with her and this may precipitate the critical event which dates the onset of disease without further question. What happens in many cases is that the patient goes out for a walk or goes shopping and cannot remember her new address. She is brought home by neighbours or the police.

Motor Restlessness

Motor restlessness is an important symptom from the diagnostic, social and medico-legal points of view. There is a locomotor restlessness which is seen in the well-known urge to wander from home. General practitioners have long recognised a group of elderly 'wanderers' although they do not identify the disease as Alzheimer's. In the literature the comical aspects of the disease at this stage in some patients have been recognised and described. In the ward the inability to sit still and the seemingly purposeful urge to rush away in a particular direction provide a caricature of the 'frightfully busy' physician suffering from a frequency of committee meetings. The patient does not know where she wants to go but does want to go somewhere. She is usually docile and if she is turned round she will walk with the same purposive air in the opposite direction. At home the elderly patient will terrify the children of the household by wandering about from room to room at night calling out for longdead relatives.

Patients in this stage of the disease are unmanageable by relatives and not suitable for admission to small private homes for the elderly. We have known instances of 'wanderers' who escaped at night and travelled miles from home before being picked up by the police.

Two other forms of restlessness deserve special comment. One form is characterised by rubbing and folding. Typically when the patient is given a newspaper to read she will spread it out on the table, fold it up, rub it smooth and continue this unfolding, folding and rubbing indefinitely. Similarly she will rub and fold a blanket, magazine, article of clothing or book. She will rub the dorsum or palm of one hand continually with the fingers of the other. A patient may produce senile purpura or even an erosion of the skin from this continual rubbing.

A second and very irritating form of compulsive activity is tapping. The patient drums on the table with her fingers, with an ash-tray or teacup. Seated in a chair she will tap her feet on the floor in a 'danse macabre'. Carphology or picking and tearing of the bed clothes is seen in the late stage of the disease. Rubbing and tapping have been observed and described by previous authors in Alzheimer's disease. We consider both movements highly characteristic as we have not observed either with certainty in any other form of disease.

Behavioural Regressions and Ideational Apraxia

The course of the disease is characterised by alterations of behaviour which make life intolerable for relatives and which determine admission to hospital in most cases. A peculiar form of gatism which we missed in early cases was noted in practically every one of our recent cases. The aberration in behaviour centres on disposal of excrement. Although it is often described as incontinence it is in fact nothing of the kind. The patient is ambulant and has sufficient control over the sphincters to go and use the chamber pot, commode or lavatory in the ordinary way. Instead of toilet paper however, she will use a handkerchief or a table napkin which she will send to the wash with other articles of clothing. She will empty the chamber pot into her own or her neighbour's garden or just downstairs. She will remove the faeces manually from bedpan or toilet and put them in a teacup, glove, handbag, her own shoe, a relative's shoe, under a pillow, sheet or mattress in her own bed or in another's bed, under the carpet or in the dust bin. In the hospital ward she will hand them to a nurse, doctor or visiting celebrity. The elderly male will empty his pipe on the electric fire, spit or urinate in the fireplace. Similarly he will get out of bed and urinate on the floor or behind a door. There is probably no other condition in which the pathological results of an organic lesion are attributed with such confidence to moral turpitude. What aggravates the delinquency is the fact that the patient is unrepentant since she cannot remember the specific incident and by reason of the amnesia she cannot learn from experience.

These deviations from the norm in social behaviour are essentially purposeful. The correct procedure has been learned in youth but has now been forgotten. As in the case of confabulation the improvised solution is faulty and socially inacceptable. A series of similar faults in behaviour can be observed in the course of the disease and are of considerable diagnostic as well as topological interest.

A very common complaint is about the patient's behaviour in regard to modern heating appliances. The elderly female will blow out the gas for example or throw rubbish on a gas or electric fire. One patient was found by her daughter on a cold day sitting in the fireplace with her head up the chimney – to keep warm as she explained! Once again we are dealing with purposeful reactions but getting further from the correct and socially acceptable procedure as the disease advances.

Another example of behavioural regression comes under the heading of ideational apraxia. A female patient was instructed in a simple task and given a ball of wool and knitting needles by the occupational therapist. Discarding the needles she managed to wind all the wool between the teeth and around the back of a large comb. She had forgotten the immediate task, forgotten the learned skill of knitting, forgotten the use of comb and knitting needles and improvised a primitive pattern of activity.

Neurological Changes

One of the earliest changes is the development of the orbicularis or so-called 'snout' reflex of WARTENBERG. If the skin below the lower lip is lightly flicked with the finger pouting of the lips occurs. WARTEN-BERG [1933] says it is particularly associated with lesions of severe cerebral degeneration in the frontal lobe. It is positive at a very early stage of Alzheimer's disease.

The sucking reflex is elicited by the examiner bringing his finger near the patient's mouth. The mouth opens to receive the finger. As an extension of this reflex, if a metallic object such as a key is offered it will be accepted and after a few moments rejected. Offered again after a brief interval it will be accepted again. This alteration in behaviour has been observed by KLÜVER and BUCY [1939] to follow destruction of the temporal lobes in monkeys. It has been described in Alzheimer's disease [PILLERI, 1961]. Judging from the severity of the lesions found *post mortem* in the hippocampus the development of the sucking reflex points to early involvement of the temporal lobe in man.

If death is not caused by intermittent disease the patient drifts into a state of general spasticity during the last few months. A grasp reflex can be demonstrated quite early in the course of the disease. The classical changes in reflexes associated with loss of upper motor neurones are well marked in the later stages of the disease. The patient is no longer ambulant. In bed she lies with her head elevated on a 'psychological pillow' for minutes at a time. This sign has been described by previous authors in other forms of senile dementia. Another type of behavioural regression is observed in the later stage when the patient tries to rise from a lying or sitting position. Instead of using the upper limbs to help she tries to get up by flexing the trunk muscles alone just as in infancy. These behavioural changes cannot be said to be characteristic of Alzheimer's disease since they are observed in other forms of chronic disease.

Defects of Speech

As might be expected from the nature and distribution of the cortical lesions defects of speech are commonly observed in the course of the disease. Stereotypy is very characteristic of the early amnesic stage. All originality is lost and the patient will not initiate a conversation. A question may be said to evoke a reflex rather than elicit a considered reply in such cases. This stereotypy is of some diagnostic value in recognising the disease at an early stage in younger subjects. Logoklonia has been regarded as a characteristic defect. It is an obtrusive form of compulsive speech which we have observed in the later stage of the disease in some cases. In the final stage the patient is completely aphasic and speech is replaced by occasional high-pitched cries reminiscent of meningitis or hydrocephalus.

Before the final stage of aphasia in some cases a very peculiar syntactic fragmentation of speech develops and is quite characteristic. We believe this is the variety of dysphasia or '*Sprachstörung*' which REDLICH described in his original case and to which there are frequent references in subsequent German literature. What happens is that in reply to a question the patient starts off with the beginning of a sentence which if ended would add up to a reasonable if stereotyped reply. A disjointed phrase could in fact be the ending or beginning of a sentence. It is an interesting variation of aphasia deriving no doubt from the complex amnesia. It is sometimes difficult to trace any relationship between the consecutive fragments of speech but it is tempting to believe that they are, or were, spatially connected in the brain.

Epileptiform Seizures

Fits deserve special mention. They were described by REDLICH even before ALZHEIMER published his account of the disease. They certainly occur in most cases and probably in every case at one time or another in the course of the disease. By reason of amnesia the patient himself does not mention them. The fit is frequently the first clinical symptom in an individual case. Relatives almost invariably refer to the episode as a 'stroke' and this prejudices medical opinion in favour of a diagnosis of cerebral vascular disease. This misinterpretation of events goes a long way to account for the neglect or missed diagnosis of Alzheimer's disease in practice. The seizures as we have observed them in hospital have all the characteristics of major epilepsy.

Tissue Atrophy

In the early stages the restless ambulant will go about the ward stealing and eating other patients' food. For the most part however she does not ask for food but eats what is offered. Later there is marked anorexia and a very severe degree of emaciation is observed in those who live long enough. This terminal emaciation in the absence of such well recognised causes as tuberculosis, cancer, diabetes, is characteristic of Alzheimer's disease. The body weight in one female went down to 30 kg before death. At *post mortem* there was a proportionate atrophy of all tissues. The brain weighed 940 g and the combined weight of both kidneys post mortem was only 165 g.

In the penultimate stage in elderly female patients, a noteworthy change develops in the facial appearance as a result of this emaciation. The superficial fat disappears and there is some wasting of the temporal muscles. The subjects appear wizened out of proportion to their chronological age and one patient tends to look remarkably like another at this stage of the illness.

Osteoporosis in Affected Males

Half way through our study we observed in a male case a severe degree of spinal osteoporosis with collapse of vertebral bodies. It was not associated with malignancy. Such a finding would not be unusual in an elderly female but this degree of osteoporosis is very unusual in a male. We therefore looked out for osteoporosis in subsequent male cases. Osteoporosis is notoriously difficult to measure and the significance of a moderate degree is difficult to assess in this age group. We found one more case of vertebral collapse in a male and moderate degree of osteoporosis of the spine in 5 out of 7 cases subsequently examined. It would be interesting if the relatively high incidence of Alzheimer's disease in women were paralleled by a high incidence of senile osteoporosis – a 'female' type of disease – in affected males.

Pathology

MCMENEMEY [1963] has provided a comprehensive account of the pathology of the disease. So much attention has been directed to the nature and significance of the individual argyrophilic lesion that we tend to overlook the really important feature of the disease which is the destruction of neural tissue. Figures for normal brain weight are notoriously difficult to obtain since so many of those in the higher age groups who come to *post mortem* are already suffering from organic cerebral disease. By accepted standards however [MCMENEMEY, 1963] in a well established case one-third of the average brain weight may be lost. Even this is an understatement of the full extent of tissue destruction. In the subject who lives long enough, functionally and structurally there is very little normal brain tissue left. To the naked eye the most important changes in the brain are the general shrinkage in size, the dilatation of the ventricles and the cortical atrophy. Histologically the enormous numbers of argyrophil plaques in the cortex form a striking and characteristic picture. There is a variety of shapes and sizes; the individual lesions range from microscopic pieces of 'Alzheimer material' up to the 'morning-star' plaque which is just visible to the naked eye in stained sections. Their distribution throughout the cortex may be quite irregular. It is generally agreed that when scarce they are most likely to be found in Ammon's horn in the temporal lobe. They are not confined to the cortex and they have been reported in the basal ganglia and corpora mammillaria. I have looked in the latter situation but have not been able to find them. NFD is a microscopic intracellular lesion. It is described in terms of tangles, baskets, loops and racquets. Granulo-vacuolar degeneration is an intracellular lesion which some observers including GRUNTHAL, GELLERSTEDT and more recently WOODARD [1967] regard as an essential histological feature of the disease. It is difficult to assess its significance at the moment and to fit in with the amyloidosis which dominates the characteristic picture of Alzheimer's disease.

As originally noted by DIVRY [1927] the Alzheimer material is birefringent and has in fact all the staining properties of amyloid. The identification has been confirmed by KIDD [1963] and TERRY [1963] who have carried out extensive studies with the electron microscope and find that the amyloid is indistinguishable from that seen in secondary amyloidosis. This must be registered as an important advance in our knowledge of the disease but the picture is still very obscure.

Amyloidosis was recognised by pathologists in the early years of the nineteenth century when it was described under the heading of lardaceous or waxy disease. According to COHEN [1967] who gives a comprehensive review of the literature, by the middle of the century VIRCHOW was able to show that the ground substance of *corpora amylacea* in the brain in old age and that of the liver in waxy disease gave the same staining reactions. Amyloidosis was known to be particularly associated with chronic infectious disease such as tuberculosis and osteomyelitis. It was also observed in horses being immunized for the production of antisera. Since the introduction of antibiotics there are fewer cases of secondary amyloidosis and interest is now focussed on these cases of amyloidosis which occur in the absence of infection.

LUBARSCH [1929] described 3 cases of 'primary' amyloidosis in middle aged subjects who were not suffering from any identifiable infectious disease. The amyloid was concentrated in unusual sites but not however in the brain. More recently there have been reports of amyloid being found widespread in the tissues of aged animals in the absence of other forms of disease.

Classification presents special problems in taxonomy and semantics. Following COHEN we can identify three major groups of morbid conditions associated with amyloidosis.

(1) A group associated with: (a) known infectious disease or (b) chronic inflammatory disease such as rheumatoid arthritis in which no infective agent has been identified. (2) A group associated with malignant disease and particularly with myelomatosis. We have seen one such case in a 60-year-old male which had many of the features of Alzheimer's disease. (3) A very large group associated with aging.

It is particularly to the last group we must look for a key to mechanism of amyloidosis in Alzheimer's disease.

Histologically amyloidosis is one of the commonest findings in aged human tissues. WALFORD and SJAARDA [1964] found amyloid in the brains of 11 out of 15 elderly subjects. According to SCHWARTZ [1967] who has found amyloid in the heart, pancreas and brain of over 80% of elderly subjects the argyrophilic lesions in the human brain correspond closely with those which take up the specific stains for amyloid.

Where the amyloidosis of Alzheimer's disease can be fitted into this picture is not yet clear. There are no less than four distinct forms of amyloid lesion in the Alzheimer brain.

(1) *Corpus amylaceum*. This lesion is found in most aged brains but the relationship with aging remains obscure. We have seen examples in Alzheimer's disease but although amyloid it is not a specific lesion. (2) *'Drüsige Entartung'* for which there is no exact English equivalent describes an amyloid degeneration of the media of the small cortical arteries. It is an intriguing lesion which some regard as an essential feature of the neuropathology of Alzheimer's disease. It appears to be identical with the medial lesions in the renal arterioles in secondary amyloidosis. SCHOLZ [1938] regarded this 'congophile angiopathy' as a characteristic lesion of Alzheimer's disease. MOREL and WILDI [1952] call it 'dyshoric angiopathy' and find it is associated with argyrophilic plaques in the senile brain. HABERLAND [1938] and VAN DER HORST [1960] have described both lesions in senile cerebral amyloidosis. (3) *Argyrophilic plaques* and (4) *Neurofibrillary degeneration* have already been described.

While amyloidosis is recognised as an immunological reaction it is also well established that it can be produced in experimental animals in the absence of infection. It is not difficult according to GAFNI *et al.* [1966] to produce amyloidosis and DRUET and JANIGAN [1966] have succeeded in producing it in mice with caseinate injections.

There is still a long way to go however before we can hope to understand the mechanism of amyloidosis in Alzheimer's disease. There is no chronic infection nor inflammatory disease, no malignant disease to which the amyloidosis might be attributed. It has been suggested [SCHWARTZ, 1965; WALFORD, 1967] that the amyloidosis of old age might be an expression of auto-immunity. If it is in fact an auto-immune reaction it is not yet clear which tissue is originally involved. Neurone, neuropil, supporting tissues and arteries are all any one of them could be the seat of the primary reaction. ...nown for some years that the brain in mongolism frequent... high concentration of plaques. It appears now that in this ...) the amyloidosis is an age related finding. In a recent series ...es going to *post mortem* OLSON and SHAW [1969] have shown ...3 subjects over the age of 35 years had neuropathological changes indistinguishable from those of Alzheimer's disease. It is difficult to arrive at any concept of mechanism which will account for the lesions in such cases. Our best guess at the moment is that the characteristic lesion in Alzheimer's disease is an auto-immune reaction involving the cortical neurones in the first instance.

The indications are that in Alzheimer's disease the earliest lesions develop in the temporal lobe and until very late in the disease they are found only in the cortex. Experimentally, therefore, it is not only a matter of inducing the specific reaction but of reproducing a topological distribution of lesions comparable to what is found in the human brain.

Identity and Diagnosis of Alzheimer's Disease

Alzheimer's is a common form of disease which can be recognised and identified with a high degree of probability on clinical grounds alone. The 'wanderer' in general practice – the ambulant aged amnesic – is almost certainly suffering from Alzheimer's disease. The cardinal symptoms are amnesia and motor restlessness. The amnesia is unlikely to be confused with Korsakoff syndromes. It is not obviously related to acute infectious disease, to alcoholism, pregnancy nor vomiting. It is progressive while the patient is still ambulant and this with negative serological tests rules out the rare case of neurosyphilis. Changes in the serum and cerebral spinal fluid are still being studied. In all our well-established cases there was a rise in serum globulin with a corresponding fall in albumin content. The present indications are that as the disease progresses there is more likely to be an increase in the a-2 globulin level in the serum.

Cerebral arteriosclerosis is the condition with which Alzheimer's disease is most often confused. Amnesia is a symptom which is common to both but whereas in Alzheimer's disease it is constant, in arteriosclerosis it can vary from day to day depending on the degree of cerebral anoxia. Focal signs are almost invariably present in cerebral arteriosclerosis and in this respect giddiness is an important sign and distinguishing feature. The early Alzheimer amnesic is restless and ambulant whilst the activity of the arteriosclerotic is more limited by a tendency to fall about.

The early changes in the facial reflexes and the behavioural regressions at this time are very characteristic and helpful in the diagnosis. So is the motor restlessness which includes ambulation, tapping, rubbing, plucking and so on. There is restlessness in the Creutzfeldt-Jakob disease but the chief movements here are clonic and involuntary. The Alzheimer movements are co-ordinated and purposive.

The EEG was abnormal in all our cases from the beginning – a finding which suggests that the disease is already advanced before clinical symptoms are recognised.

The clinical syndrome is to be distinguished from other forms of dementia which occur in old age and at this end of the spectrum from normal aging. In extreme old age there may be amnesia and dementia associated with an extensive fall out of neurones and loss of brain weight *post mortem*. In such case it may be difficult to assess the significance of a small number of plaques. The provenance and fate of the amyloid plaque remain obscure. The amyloid must disappear in the course of time. We can never be quite certain therefore that the plaques seen confirm the nature or reflect the severity of the disease. We noted particularly after a cortical biopsy in two of our cases there was some clinical improvement. One could envisage a situation in which plaque formation ceased for a time and the existing amyloid was dissipated.

The relationship with aging is complex. Aging is a vague concept incapable of exact definition. Above all it is an abstract term and as such cannot be the cause of any disease. The basis of Alzheimer's disease is an age-related amyloidosis. This can begin at any age if the essential causative factors operate but why they should tend to operate at a later rather than an earlier age in a given case we do not know.

Something occurs after cerebral trauma [McMenemey, 1963] and in mongolism which triggers off the reaction at an earlier date. The observations of Olson and Shaw [1969] suggest that if a mongol lives long enough he must develop Alzheimer's disease and there is much to suggest that the same holds good for the normal human being. The statement that plaques are found in normal subjects is one which begs many questions. The plaque is always pathological but the finding of a few plaques in an otherwise normal brain will not label the case one of Alzheimer's disease.

263

McMenemey [1963] from the neuropathological standpoint regards the generic condition as one of cerebral amyloidosis in which Alzheimer's disease is subsumed with other specific entities including certain cases of Pick's disease, Simmond's disease, neurosyphilis and the rare cases which follow cerebral trauma. From this approach the diagnosis of Alzheimer's disease would still rest on clinical criteria in the first instance. We consider that the name should be reserved for cases in which a pattern of symptoms such as we have described has evolved during life. For the reasons stated above the diagnosis should not be restricted to those cases in which a high concentration of plaques is found *post mortem*.

Sim [1965] pleads for a wider recognition of Alzheimer's disease – the 'forgotten entity'. For its economic importance alone it certainly deserves more attention. From an academic approach we know of no other disease which provides such interesting material for the analysis of human behaviour. In the individual case we are witnessing the disintegration of integration. The dysphasia presents us with new ideas of concepts. The amnesia sets us thinking about our basic knowledge of knowledge and understanding of understanding.

It is true that up to now the prognosis is hopeless but with the newer interest in amyloidosis the position may change. We support Sim's plea for its recognition as a very important disease.

Summary

Alzheimer's disease is a common form of disease of the elderly which accounts for the occupancy of up to a fifth of our geriatric beds. In a confused nomenclature it is frequently called senile psychosis or senile dementia both of which terms are used to cover unrelated forms of disease. This has led to a neglect of the disease which is rarely recognised although it can be diagnosed with near certainty on clinical grounds alone. The pathological basis is cerebral amyloidosis. The indications are that this is an expression of age-related auto-immunity. As a study in the disintegration of behaviour Alzheimer's disease presents problems of absorbing interest.

References

Alzheimer, A.: Über eine eigenartige Erkrankung der Hirnrinde. Allg. Z. Psychiat. *64:* 146–148 (1907).
Cohen, A. S.: Amyloidosis. New Engl. J. Med. *277:* 522–530, 574–583, 628–638 (1967).
Divry, P. et Florkin, M.: Sur les propriétés de l'amyloïde. Comptes rend. Soc. biol. *97:* 1808–1810 (1927).

Druet, R. L. and Janigan, D. T.: Experimental amyloidosis. Amer. J. Path. *49:* 1103–1124 (1966).

Fischer, O.: Die presbyophrene Demenz. Z. ges. Neurol. Psychiat. *3:* 371–470 (1910).

Gafni, J.; Merker, H. J.; Shibolet, S.; Sohar, E. and Heller, H.: On the origin of amyloid. Amer. int. Med. *65:* 1031–1043 (1906).

Gellerstedt, M.: Zur Kenntnis der Hirnveränderungen bei normaler Altersinvolution. Arbeiten aus dem pathologischen Institut. Upsala LäkFören. Förh. *38:* 193–408 (1933).

Grünthal, E.: Über die Alzheimerische Krankheit. Z. ges. Neurol. Psychiat. *101:* 128–157 (1926).

Haberland, C.: Primary systematic amyloidosis. J. Neuropath. exp. Neurol. *23:* 135–150 (1964).

Horst, van der, L.; Stam, F. C. and Wigdobolus, J. M.: Amyloidosis in senile and presenile involutional processes of the central nervous system. J. nerv. ment. Dis. *130:* 578–587 (1960).

Kidd, M.: Paired helical filaments in electron microscopy of Alzheimer's disease. Nature, Lond. *197:* 192–193 (1963).

Klüver, H. and Bucy, P. C.: Preliminary analysis of functions of temporal lobes in monkeys. Arch. Neurol. Psychiat. *42:* 979–983 (1939).

Lhermitte, J. et Nicolas: La démence sénile et ses formes anatomocliniques. Encéphale *19:* 583–594, 654–665 (1924).

Lubarsch, O.: Zur Kenntnis ungewöhnlicher Amyloidablagerungen. Virchows Arch. path. Anat. *271:* 867–889 (1929).

McMenemey, W. H.: Greenfield's Neuropathology (London 1963).

Morel, F. and Wildi, E.: Proceedings First International Congress of Neuropathology *II:* 347 (1952).

Newton, R. D.: The identity of Alzheimer's disease and senile dementia and their relationship to senility. J. ment. Sci. *94:* 225–249 (1948).

Olson, M. I. and Shaw, C. M.: Dementia in mongolism. Brain *92:* 147–156 (1969).

Pilleri, G.: Orale Einstellung nach Art des Klüver Bucy Syndroms bei hirnatrophischen Prozessen. Schweiz. Arch. Neurol. Neurochir. Psychiat. *87:* 286–298 (1961).

Redlich, E.: Über miliare Sklerose der Hirnrinde bei seniler Atrophie. J. Psychiat. Neurol. *17:* 208–216 (1898).

Rothschild, D.: Pathological changes in senile psychoses and their psychological significance. Amer. J. Psychiat. *93:* 757–788 (1937).

Scholz, W.: Die drüsige Entartung der Hirnarterien und Kapillaren. Z. ges. Neurol. Psychiat. *162:* 695–715 (1938).

Schwartz, D.: Senile cerebral, pancreatic insular and cardiac amyloidosis. Trans. N.Y. Acad. Sci. *27:* 393–413 (1965).

Simchowitz, T.: Histologische Studien über die senile Demenz. Hist. Histopathol. Arb. Nissl. *4:* 268–273 (1910).

Simchowitz, T.: La maladie d'Alzheimer et son rapport avec la démence sénile. Encéphale *9:* 218–231 (1914).

Terry, R. D.: Fine structure of neurofibrillary tangles in Alzheimer's disease. J. Neuropath. exp. Neurol. *22:* 629–642 (1963).

Walford, R. L.: Advances in Gerontological Research (New York 1967).

Walford, R. L. and Sjaarda, J. R.: Increase of thioflavine – T-staining material (amyloid) in human tissues with age. J. Geront. *19:* 57–61 (1964).

Wartenberg, R.: Diagnostic Tests in Neurology (Chicago 1953).

Woodard, J. S.: Alzheimer's disease in later adult life. Amer. J. Path. *49:* 1157–1165 (1966).

AUTHOR INDEX

KEY-WORD TITLE INDEX

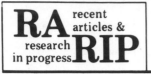

RA recent articles &
research RIP
in progress

Guide to Current Research

The research summaries appearing in the following section were obtained through a search of the Smithsonian Science Information Exchange data base conducted in November, 1973.

The Exchange annually registers 85,000 to 100,000 notices of current research projects covering a wide range of disciplines and sources of support. SSIE endeavors to retain up to two full years of current research information in its active file. The selection of summaries appearing in this section does not represent the complete SSIE collection of information on this topic, but, rather, has been specifically tailored to reflect the scientific content of this particular volume. A limited number of summaries may have been omitted because clearance for publication by the supporting agency or organization was not received prior to the publication date.

SSIE is the only, single source for information on ongoing and recently terminated research in all areas of the life, physical, behavioral, social and engineering sciences. The SSIE file is updated daily by a professional staff of scientists utilizing a comprehensive and flexible system of hierarchical indexing. Retrieval of subject information is conducted by these same specialists, using computer-connected, video display terminals which allow instant access to the entire data base and on-line refinement of search strategies. SSIE offers an information service unequalled anywhere: comprehensive and vital information on who is conducting what research where and under whose support.

More current information, and in some cases expanded coverage, on the topic considered in this volume is available directly from SSIE. This information is offered at modest cost in the form of custom searches of the SSIE file designed specifically to meet the user's need or as an update of the subject search in this section. For more information on SSIE, contact MSS or write directly to the Smithsonian Science Information Exchange, 1730 M Street, N.W., Washington, D.C. 20036. Subject search or updated package requirements may be discussed with SSIE scientists by calling the Exchange at (202) 381-5511.

STUDIES IN AGEING OF THE BRAIN,
J.H. AUSTIN, Univ. of Colorado, School of
Medicine, Denver, Colorado 80220

These studies are designed to clarify
the relationships between Alzheimer's
disease and conventional ageing of the
brain.
Changes in silicon levels in various
tissues and body fluids are also under
investigation both in humans and
experimental animals.

SUPPORTED BY:
U.S. Dept. of Hlth. Ed. & Wel. - N.I.H.

REGULATION OF REGIONAL INTRACEREBRAL
CIRCULATION DURING INJURY AND AGING,
J.N. BARKER, New York University, School of
Medicine, New York, New York 10016

Objectives: The goals of this project
are to: 1. learn the local distribution of
brain flow in normal and pathologic
conditions and the factors which contribute
to its maldistribution at normal flow rates
in rats; 2. devise methods for measurements
in man and the correction of the
cerebrovascular insufficiencies occurring in
localized regions of the brain.
Methodology: 1. Local blood flow is
measured by the C14 antipyrine uptake method
with direct analysis of microdissected
regions. 2. S35 and Se75 methionine uptake
are used as a measure of local metabolic
activity. 3. All aged rats are studied at
some stage of aging or disease of particular
interest. 4. Xe133 uptake as a measure of
blood flow and Se75 monitoring as a measure
of metabolism can be used to observe changes
in parameters of the living animal. 5.

More than 100 rats have been studied; about
40 are being aged or are in process of being
analyzed. Several hundred regions of
special interest are examined in each brain.

Results: 1. The study was expanded
this year to devise the method by which both
metabolism and blood flow could be monitored
in vivo. This method shows excellent
correlation with clinical condition of the
animal. 2. Progress in learning how some
forms of local cerebrovascular
insufficiencies arise and produce conditions
which increase susceptibility to stroke of
the hyperperfusion and hypoperfusion types
has been made. 3. Shunting phenomena with
the cortex and layers of it have been
confirmed. The absolute rates of cortical
flow can vary from less than half normal to
twice normal. The cortex, especially the
parietal region, shows such wide flow
variations that it is likely to have been
designed to dampen brief flow transients,
thereby protecting vital deeper structures.
Inside the basal ganglia, the caudate
nucleus appears to perform a similar
function, especially when flow is slowed.

SUPPORTED BY:
U.S. Dept. of Hlth. Ed. & Wel. - S.R.S.

ELECTRON MICROSCOPY AND NEUROCHEMISTRY OF
THE BRAIN IN AGING,
A. BIGNAMI, U.S. Veterans Administration,
Hospital, Palo Alto, California 94304

Differentiation of Astrocytes.
Immunofluorescence study with Antibodies to
the Glial Fibrillary Acidic Protein (GFAP),
A Brain Specific Protein in Astrocytic Blia
(Bignami and Dahl, Brain Research, in
press): In the cerebellar cortex of the
newborn rat immunofluorescent astrocytic

fibers appear on the 4th postnatal day and acquire their adult shape at the end of the second week, suggesting that they may play a role in directing neuronal migration. In the pyramidal tracts, they are first observed when myelination starts, suggesting the simultaneous differentiation of oligodendroglia and astroglia. Biochemical Study of Rat Optic Nerves in Wallerian Degeneration (Bignami and Eng, J. Neurochem., in press): With the exception of ethanolamineglycerophosphatide, there is no preferential breakdown of myelin lipid or protein in Wallerian degeneration. Purification of GFAP From Normal Human Brain (Dahl and Bignami, submitted for publication): GFAP was previously obtained from enriched material (glial scars). It has now been purified from normal human brain, allowing the use of more readily available material and permitting comparative studies in pathological conditions and aging. GFAP in Philogenesis (Dahl and Bignami, in preparation): Proteins sharing common antigenic determinants with human GFAP are present in the CNS of all vertebrates, the lamprey excluded. However, the optic nerves of the goldfish and frog which possess remarkable regenerative capacities following transection do not possess GFAP. We are interested in this work because of the possibility that the glia scar is the main factor preventing regeneration in the CNS.

SUPPORTED BY:
U.S. Veterans Administration

REACTIONS OF OXIDIZED LIPIDS WITH PROTEINS,
K.L. CARRAWAY, Okla. St. Univ., School of
Agriculture, Stillwater, Oklahoma 74075

This project will focus upon the
chemistry involved in the reactions of
oxidized unsaturated lipids with proteins
with the goal of clarifying the importance
of these reactions to degenerative processes
in biological systems. Three different
systems will be studied: 1) the reaction of
oxidized lipids and their products with
amino acids, 2) the reaction of oxidized
lipids and their products with proteins and
3) the oxidation of a model cell membrane
system. The purpose of the three systems
are, respectively, 1) to determine the
nature of the products which result from the
reaction of the amino acid side chains of
proteins with oxidized lipids, 2) to
determine the reactions and factors which
are important in destruction of enzyme
activities and crosslinking of proteins by
oxidized lipids, and 3) to develop this
knowledge for use in analyzing tissue or
cell components involved in oxidative
deterioration. The chemical and physical
properties of the crosslinked products of
proteins and membranes will be studied in an
effort to obtain parameters by which these
materials can be compared to the lipofuchsin
pigments and similar products of oxidative
deterioration which arise during the course
of aging, atherosclerosis and similar
degenerative diseases. Of particular
interest is the susceptibility of these
various crosslinked products to enzymic
degradation, since a low rate of natural
enzymic degradation may account for the
accumulation of these materials within the
cell. Additional research into the nature
of the lipofuchsin pigments will then be
pursued using methods developed for the

study of products of reactions of proteins
and oxidized lipids.

SUPPORTED BY:
U.S. Dept. of Hlth. Ed. & Wel. - N.I.H.

ELECTRON MICROSCOPY OF BONE AND SKELETAL
MUSCLE,
R.R. COOPER, Univ. of Iowa, School of
Medicine, Iowa City, Iowa 52240

     During this research project, I want to
delineate ultrastructural morphology of bone
as an organ and as a tissue in humans and
animals during normal growth, development,
and aging and to describe variations of
normal growth produced by experiment and
disease. I will correlate these studies
with light microscopic and biochemical
examination of the same tissues. This
includes examination of nerve supply of bone
as a function of age; determination of the
type of nerve endings in bone; examination
of ligament and tendon insertions as related
to age, experiment, and disease; examination
of epiphysis and epiphyseal plate
development in normal animals and humans,
and during epiphyseal growth and
developmental disorders.
     I want to determine microscopic,
ultrastructural, electrical and mechanical
changes in cat skeletal muscle during disuse
and denervation atrophy and during
regeneration after disuse. I want to
compare these findings with biopsies of
human neuromuscular disease. I hope also to
delineate the normal ultrastructural
morphology of muscle spindles.

SUPPORTED BY:
U.S. Dept. of Hlth. Ed. & Wel. - N.I.H.

CHANGES IN THE EXCITABILITY CYCLE OF THE
VISUAL EVOKED RESPONSE DURING AGING,
R.E. DUSTMAN, U.S. Veterans Administration,
Hospital, Salt Lake City, Utah 84113

We have recorded the evoked responses
of approximately 50 elderly subjects to
single stimuli. Data from these subjects
support earlier findings with geriatric
subjects in that early evoked response waves
occur later and are larger than these waves
are in the responses of younger subjects.
We have recently written computer
programs which will enable us to randomly
present single and pairs of stimuli during a
recording session and to sum responses to
each. We will thus have an evoked response
to single stimuli to compare with responses
to paired stimuli with both having been
recorded during identical conditions of
background EEG, alertness, etc.
Interstimulus intervals for the paired
stimuli will be selected to enable us to
determine the relationship of the late
positive-negative wave (peaking at about
140 msec.) to cortical excitability.

SUPPORTED BY:
U.S. Veterans Administration

SENESCENT VISUAL AND SOMATOSENSORY EVOKED
RESPONSES - A COMPARATIVE STUDY,
R.E. DUSTMAN, U.S. Veterans Administration,
Hospital, Salt Lake City, Utah 84113

Of the original group of geriatric
patients studied, patients in three
diagnostic classifications were selected:
arteriosclerosis; chronic brain syndrome,
alcoholism. Ns were 18, 8, and 6
respectively. The visual, auditory, and

somatosensory evoked responses of these
patients were compared on the basis of
amplitude and peak delay with those of
age-matched normal subjects.

Many statistically significant results
were found differentiating patients from
normals and suggest that the evoked response
may be helpful in differentially identifying
various clinical conditions.

SUPPORTED BY:
U.S. Veterans Administration

BRAIN CATECHOLAMINES AND AGING,
C.E. FINCH, Univ. of Southern California,
Graduate School, Los Angeles, California
90007

This research program has been
concerned with determining the endocrine and
autonomic function in mammals. Because the
seats of endocrine and autonomic control lie
within the brain, the research has examined
the effects of aging in cell function in
relevant brain regions (hypothalamus, limbic
system, and brain stem) by studies of
protein synthesis and catecholamine
metabolism; these studies will be continued.
The effects of aging on pituitary hormones
and hypothalamic releasing factors, about
which little is known at present, will also
be examined.

SUPPORTED BY:
U.S. Natl. Science Foundation

GENE FUNCTION DURING POST-NATAL DEVELOPMENT
AND AGING,
C.E. FINCH, Univ. of Southern California,
Gerontology Center, Los Angeles, California
90007

Cellular differentiation will be measured at critical stages of post-natal development and aging in terms of nuclear gene-transcription with techniques of RNA-DNA hybridization. Study of transcription in brain regions may lead to identification of pacemakers of aging. Examination of reassociation kinetics of sheared DNA from young and old rodent neurones (non-dividing cells) and livers (dividing cells) will test the theory that there is a significant accumulation of cross-links in DNA during aging.

SUPPORTED BY:
U.S. Dept. of Hlth. Ed. & Wel. - N.I.H.

GABA METABOLISM--A BIOCHEMICAL KEY TO MENTAL AGING,
M.L. FONDA, Univ. of Louisville, School of Medicine, Louisville, Kentucky 40202

In this study the relationship of gamma-aminobutyrate (GABA) and its metabolism to biological aging is being investigated. The steady state concentration of the metabolites and enzymes of the GABA metabolic pathway is being determined in brain tissue of individual mice of known biological ages, including senescent.

Specific inhibitors of purified brain glutamate decarboxylase and GABA-aminotransferase, enzymes that control the brain level of GABA, will be investigated. These specific inhibitors and compounds which either block or prolong the neurochemical action of GABA will be investigated as possible means of controlling the in vivo concentration of GABA in mice of different biological ages.

SUPPORTED BY:
U.S. Dept. of Hlth. Ed. & Wel. - N.I.H.

NEUROENDOCRINE AND BEHAVIORAL CORRELATES OF
AGING,
S.E. HENDRICKS, Univ. of Nebraska, School of
Liberal Arts, Omaha, Nebraska 68132

The broad aim of the project is to
specify the role of neuroendocrine systems
in the development and aging of an organism.
Behavioral measures over age and in response
to various manipulations affecting the
neuroendocrine system are the primary
dependent variables being used. Sexual
behavior is being particularly emphasized.
However, operant behaviors, activity levels,
and other behaviors are also being studied.
Additionally, some morphological changes in
the central nervous system which occur in
response to hormonal manipulations during
prenatal and neonatal life are being
studied. The possibility that these same or
similar changes occur with maturation and
aging is also to be investigated.

SUPPORTED BY:
U.S. Dept. of Hlth. Ed. & Wel. - N.I.H.

SPECIFIC DNA CHANGES IN AGING,
R.L. HERRMANN, U.S. Veterans Administration,
Hospital, Bedford, Massachusetts 01867

Age-related changes have been observed
in rapidly reassociating DNA fractions from
C57BL/6 mouse liver and brain. In addition,
a hitherto unknown DNA fraction, which
reassociates spontaneously and has a

hairpin-like structure, has been isolated which increases two-fold in old animals. A paper reporting these results was recently submitted to Biochimica et Biophysica Acta. We propose to extend these studies by physical and chemical analysis of the DNA fractions and by the study of other aging tissues. Our overall hypothesis considers the possibility that the changes in these isolated DNA fractions may portend an alteration in the mammalian genome such that gene sequences are progressively lost from the information content of the cells.

Isolated DNA fractions are presently being characterized by enzymatic digestion with the proteolytic enzyme pronase, with nucleases DNase and RNase and the endonuclease from wheat seedlings. Spectral measurements of these fractions are also being carried out with the help of Dr. Anthony Russell in this laboratory. We also plan to examine the protein content with an amino acid analyzer and the structure by further electron microscopic studies presently being carried out in the laboratory of Dr. Charles Thomas at Harvard Medical School. We are also examining non-differentiating tissues to attempt to exclude the possibility that the observed changes are a part of normal tissue differentiation.

Our long rang goals envision attempts to alter the production of these structures by means of drug therapy with the expectation that the possible age-related degeneration of the genome may be prevented and the useful life span extended.

SUPPORTED BY:
U.S. Veterans Administration

REACTICNS OF OXIDIZED LIPIDS WITH PRCTEINS,
J.W. HUGGINS, Okla. St. Univ., School of
Agriculture, Stillwater, Oklahoma 74075

This project will focus upon the
chemistry involved in the reactions cf
oxidized unsaturated lipids with proteins
with the goal of clarifying the importance
of these reactions to degenerative processes
in biclogical systems. Three different
systems will be studied: 1) the reaction of
oxidized lipids and their products with
amino acids, 2) the reaction of oxidized
lipids and their products with proteins and
3) the oxidaticn of a model cell membrane
system. The purpose of the three systems
are, respectively, 1) to determine the
nature of the products which results frcm
the reaction of the amino acid side chains
cf proteins with oxidized lipids, 2) to
determine the reactions and factors which
are important in destruction of enzyme
activities and crosslinking of proteins by
oxidized lipids, and 3) to develop this
knowledge for use in analyzing tissue or
cell ccmponents involved in oxidative
deterioration. The chemical and physical
properties of the crosslinked products of
proteins and membranes will be studied in an
effort to obtain parameters by which these
materials can be compared tc the lipofuchsin
pigments and similar products of oxidative
deterioration which arise during the course
of aging, atherosclerosis and similar
degenerative diseases. Of particular
interest is the susceptibility of these
various crosslinked products to enzymic
degradation, since a low rate of natural
enzymic degradation may acccunt for the
accumulation of these materials within the
cell. Additional research into the nature
of the lipofuchsin pigments will then be
pursued using methods developed for the

study of products of reactions of proteins
and oxidized lipids.

SUPPORTED BY:
Oklahoma Heart Association

BRAIN 2-HYDROXY FATTY ACID METABOLISM AND
MYELINATION,

Y. KISHIMOTO, E.K. Shriver Ctr. Mental Ret.,
Waltham, Massachusetts 02154

This program is focused on the study of
enzyme systems for the biosynthesis and
oxidative decarboxylation of 2-hydroxy fatty
acids in the brain. In recent preliminary
experiments, we have for the first time
demonstrated the in vitro biosynthesis of
brain 2-hydroxy fatty acid. We will attempt
to solubilize, purify, and characterize
these enzymes. The effects of various
controlling factors, such as aging,
hormones, and drugs will be studied. We
will attempt to separate the enzyme which
converts 2-hydroxy fatty acids to 2-keto
acids from that which catalyzes further
oxidative decarboxylation. The unique
features of the assay for 2-hydroxy acid
biosynthesis in this proposal are: (1) use
of 1-C14-lignoceric acid which is the major
natural substrate of the enzyme and which we
believe, therefore, has more affinity for
the enzyme than the commonly available
1-C14-stearic acid, (2) use of the copper
chelate for isolation of the enzymically
formed cerebronic acid (2- hydroxy
lignoceric acid). For the investigation of
oxidative decarboxylation of 2-hydroxy
acids, 1-C14-cerebronic acid will be used as
the substrate and evolved 14CO2 will be
collected. To assay 2-keto acid formation
from 2-hydroxy acid, TLC fractionation or
Girard reagent extraction will be employed.

2-hydroxy acids are primarily myelin
components. The relationship between their
metabolism and myelination will be
investigated by two approaches: (1)
experimental delay in myelination will be
produced in developing animals by (a)
neonatal hypothyroidism, (b) neonatal
hyperphenylalanemia, (c) undernutrition,
and (d) neonatal X-ray irradiation. The
metabolism of brain 2-hydroxy acid will be
studied in these animals. If drugs such as
phenobarbital are found to induce the
2-hydroxylation of brain fatty acids, we
will examine if these drugs can, in part,
counteract the delay of myelination in these
experimental animals; (2) we will
investigate the effect of an inhibitor of
the enzyme for 2-hydroxy acid synthesis on
myelination in cultured peripheral nerve
cells.

SUPPORTED BY:
U.S. Dept. of Hlth. Ed. & Wel. - N.I.H.

ROLE OF BIOLOGICAL MEMBRANES IN AGING
PROCESSES,
E.J. MASORO, Medical Coll. of Pennsylvania,
School of Medicine, Philadelphia,
Pennsylvania 19129

The overall objective of this program
project research is to evaluate the role of
altered membrane structure and function in
the aging process. Membranes are focused
upon because of their prime position in
integration and regulation of metabolism and
thus most physiological activities.
Specifically the relationships between
possible alterations in membrane structure
and function during aging to several aspects
of muscle and nervous tissue function will
be investigated. 1) The exploration of the
molecular basis for the deficiency of muscle

function in the aged will be pursued by the
following approaches: a) Investigations of
possible alterations of excitable membranes
of muscle during aging will be made. b)
Investigations of possible alterations of
sarcoplasmic reticulum membranes during
aging with particular emphasis on the
processes of excitation-contraction coupling
and muscle relaxation will be carried out.
c) Investigation on possible alterations in
the contractile proteins (actin and myosin)
and the modulating proteins (troponin and
tropomyosin) during aging will be made. 2)
The exploration of possible reasons for
neurophysiologic deficiencies which occur
during aging will be done by making
measurements on action potential coding
patterns and metabolic activities of neurons
at a cortical level. These measurements
will provide information on the excitable
membranes of neurons, the synaptic membranes
and the stimulus-metabolic transduction
potentialities of the system.

SUPPORTED BY:
U.S. Dept. of Hlth. Ed. & Wel. - N.I.H.

FATTY ACID METABOLISM IN TOCOPHEROL
DEFICIENCY,
P.B. MCCAY, Univ. of Oklahoma, School of
Medicine, Oklahoma City, Oklahoma 73104

     Results of our investigations have
shown that the activity of the microsomal
TPNH oxidase system (and other
oxido-reductase systems) is accompanied by
the production of a factor having the
properties of a free radical. This factor
appears to be responsible for the chemical
alteration of constituent phospholipids in
the microsomal membrane, which we had

established earlier as being a consequence
of electron transport by the TPNH-dependent
system. The alteration consists of a
multiple peroxidative chain cleavage of the
beta-position polyunsaturated fatty acids in
the phospholipids and leads to the
accumulation of phospholipids with
carbonyl-containing fatty acyl groups in the
beta-position. The result is a decrease in
the polyunsaturated fatty acid content of
the microsome and a measurable change in the
physical properties of this membranous
organelle. Microsomal alpha- tocopherol is
consumed during the initial part of the
reaction. The studies support the
hypothesis that certain oxido-reductase
systems produce potentially damaging
radicals in the mechanism of their action
and that alpha-tocopherol functions to limit
the extent of such damage at a level
required to maintain cellular integrity.
The capacity of other structurally unrelated
compounds with free radical trapping
proportion to substitute for dietary
alpha-tocopherol may be explained by these
results. The further objectives of this
study are to obtain additional evidence that
the activity of membrane-bound electron
transport systems is responsible for the
membrane damage observed to occur when
animals are fed diets containing inadequate
levels of alpha- tocopherol or other free
radical-trapping agents. The extent to
which such damage can disrupt functions of
the endoplasmic reticulum such as protein
synthesis and the metabolic turnover of
polyenoic fatty acids in this structure is
also an objective. In addition, the
possibility that the enzyme-dependent
peroxidative chain cleavage of phospholipids
promotes the formation of lipofuscin
pigments in certain disease states, and in
tocopherol-deficient and aging animals will
be evaluated.

SUPPORTED BY:
U.S. Dept. of Hlth. Ed. & Wel. - N.I.H.

THE ALPHA-OXIDATION SYSTEM OF THE BRAIN,
J.F. MEAD, Univ. of California, Lab. of
Nucl. Med. Rad. Biol., Los Angeles,
California 90024

The objective of this research is to
characterize the enzymes involved in the
Alpha-oxidation system of the brain
microsomes and to determine the function of
this system in brain metabolism and
function. The importance of the system stems
from the finding that its products appear to
increase during aging and that it may
represent the only means by which the brain
can degrade the potentially toxic very
long-chain fatty acids released during
demyelination or other degradative
processes.
Since the reaction has been shown to
take place in live animals, the present
effort is to characterize the enzyme in
vitro, in preparations from brains of rats
and other animals. In general, the second
step of the reaction, decarboxylation of the
long-chain Alpha- hydroxy acids, has been
studied using $C14-$ or $H3$-labeled substrates.
Results: The results to date have
shown that the enzyme is present in the
brain "microsomal" fraction and that $Fe2$
ion, oxygen and the 100,000xg cell
supernatant fraction are required. The
supernatant fraction can be substituted by
ascorbic acid and scorbutic guinea pigs have
very low Alpha-oxidation rates.

SUPPORTED BY:
U.S. Atomic Energy Commission

A STUDY OF NORMAL AND DISEASED EXTRAOCULAR
MUSCLE,
J.E. MILLER, Washington University, School
of Medicine, Saint Louis, Missouri 63110

It is planned to investigate
extraocular and other muscles from humans,
monkeys, and lower animals. The influence
of aging, thyroid disease, strabismus
surgery, nerve section, and central nervous
system lesions will be evaluated.
Investigation is to continue in an
attempt to categorize the muscle fibers in
extrinsic eye muscle and to associate the
types of motor end plates and nerves that
innervate each fiber.
It is also planned to relate the types
of muscle cells to different forms of eye
movement by inducing chronic brain lesions
and evaluating the histologic change within
the muscle.

SUPPORTED BY:
U.S. Dept. of Hlth. Ed. & Wel. - N.I.H.

PLASMA PROTEIN ELECTROPHORETIC PATTERN AND
BLOOD VISCOSITY IN ARTERIOSCLEROTIC CHRONIC
BRAIN SYNDROME,
S.A. MRAZEK, U.S. Veterans Administration,
Center, Biloxi, Mississippi 39531

Fifty-one male patients who have been
in a Veterans Administration
neuropsychiatric hospital for an average of
almost 13 years underwent clinical and
laboratory examinations to determine the
degree of change in their condition since
the last admission. The average age was 63
years (range, 29-88). No consistent
abnormalities were noted in blood viscosity,
serum calcium or serum cholesterol.

Although urinary 17- ketosteroid excretion
was not related to age, it was related (low
excretion) to osteoporosis. Plasma protein
electrophoresis showed no relation between
total lipoproteins and age. However, there
was much greater variability of the alpha
globulin fractions in patients over 63 years
of age. Chronic brain syndrome (chiefly
associated with cerebral arteriosclerosis)
became the predominant diagnosis after age
63.

SUPPORTED BY:
U.S. Veterans Administration

ROLE OF ATTENTION IN MOTOR MECHANISMS,
J.H. PETAJAN, U.S. Veterans Administration,
Hospital, Salt Lake City, Utah 84113

The ability to sustain the firing of a
single motor unit in first dorsal
interosseous muscle utilizing audio-visual
feedback of the motor unit action potential
is being determined in subjects of varying
ages. Feedback is required to sustain the
firing of only a single motor unit. A
computer program utilizing the PDP-9
computer has been developed to characterize
the duration and periodicity of lapses in
firing. This program is now being used to
verify findings obtained in a group of 25
adult subjects. The periodicity of lapses
for this group averaged ten times per minute
for motor units that lapsed (type II).
Another type of unit (type I) encountered
less frequently rarely lapses, lapses
occurring only one to three times per
minute. Units that lapse frequently require
insistent reactivation; firing is not
automatic. Sustained attention is required
to keep these units firing. For motor units
that fire with few lapses, less effort or
attention is required to sustain their

firing. From these observations it is clear
that two types of motor can be distinguished
purely on the basis of the tendency to
lapse. In terms of the attention mechanism
involved required to sustain firing, cyclic
(or short term) and tonic (or automatic)
types of mechanisms seem to be involved.

Adolescent subjects are being compared
with elderly (7C plus years) subjects. The
young subjects do not differ significantly
from the adult group. However, without
exception no tonic (or automatic) units
(type II) have been found in four elderly
subjects. These findings suggest the
requirement for insistent reactivation of
motor unit firing to sustain minimal effort
in the elderly. It suggests as a basis for
senile tremor the loss of small tonic
motoneurons. The extent to which the
intrinsic hand muscles reflect the cortical
activation of motoneurons in this instance
may indicate a corresponding alteration in
attention mechanism occurring in old age.

SUPPORTED BY:
U.S. Veterans Administration

ANALYSIS CF GENETIC EFFECTS ON AGING,
E.S. RUSSELL, Roscoe B. Jackson Mem. Lab.,
Bar Harbor, Maine 04609

This program consists of six specific
projects dealing with aging of genetically
controlled laboratory mice. Dr. Myers will
determine total lifespans and incidence of
pathology in C57BL/6, DEA/2, B5D2F1, CBA/Ca,
and CBA/H-T6/T6 mice, with modern
clean-conventional husbandry. Dr. Sprott
will delineate age-dependent behavioral
changes in C57BL/6, DBA/2, and B6D2F1 mice,
study the roles of genotype and past
experience in controlling behavioral

changes, and determine effects of
long-lasting behavior patterns on longevity.
 Dr. Eleftheriou will evaluate
neurochemical, neuroendocrine, and
neurophysiological status of aging C57BL/6,
DBA/2, and B6D2F1 mice, including changes in
five specific regions of the brain and
systemic endocrine changes. Dr. Harrison
will investigate possible aging changes in
the number and proliferative capacity of
hemopoietic stem cells of C57BL/6, DBA/2,
B6D2F1 and CBA mice. Drs. Murphy and
Russell will determine how mutant alleles at
the W-locus shorten lifespan through primary
gene effects limited to hemopoietic tissue
and gonads, using intergenotype
transplantation between (C57BL/6 x
C3H)F1-Wx/Wv anemic sterile and congenic
plus/plus normal mice.

SUPPORTED BY:
U.S. Dept. of Hlth. Ed. & Wel. - N.I.H.

VASCULAR STUDIES OF WORKERS EXPOSED TO
CARBON DISULFIDE,
 SAVIC, Inst. of Occup. & Radiol. Hlth,
Belgrade, Yugoslavia

     Besides the neurotropic effects of CS2
it recently has been reported that vascular
changes also occur. The angiotropic effects
of CS2 were reported primarily for the
arteries of the brain and appear as
arteriolo-and arteriosclerotic changes which
were implicated in the neurologic changes.
It has also been shown that workers with
long exposures to CS2 have microaneurisms in
the retinal blood vessels. Changes in
carbohydrate and lipoprotein metabolism also
have been observed in CS2 intoxication. It

is possible that these metabolic and histological changes are related. It should be pointed out however, that these later observations were made exclusively on older workers in whom sclerotic and metabolic changes would be quite prevalent.

The objectives of this study are to determine the relationship of the vascular lesions to the level and duration of carbon disulfide exposure and age of worker; which of the lesions are primary (vascular or neurologic); whether the neurologic and vascular lesions are independent or interrelated; whether the vascular changes in chronic CS2 exposure are the same as those in diabetes mellitus and aging; the value of vascular changes in the early recognition and diagnosis of chronic, low level, subclinical CS2 intoxication; to differentiate vascular changes in CS2 exposure from those of low level lead exposure hypothyroidism, and aging.

SUPPORTED BY:
U.S. Dept. of Hlth. Ed. & Wel. - H.S.M.H.A

COMPARATIVE NEUROLOGY AND NEUROPATHOLOGY OF ATAXIC MICE,
D.S. SAX, U.S. Veterans Administration, Hospital, Boston, Massachusetts 02130

The Comparative Neurology Laboratory has continued to develop the studies as outlined in the protocol. There has been a delay in the electronmicroscopy aspects of fine structural analysis because of the unexpected departure of the electronmicroscopist, and the subsequent closing down of the EM Lab. Light microscopy and autoradiographic analysis of the mutant strains in mice was continued. Specimens were prepared for ultrastructural analysis.

Further definition of the hydrocephalus seen in the quaking strain as well as in the staggerer was obtained. It appears that the hydrocephalus is related to: (1) nutritional status; (2) artifact of fixation, due to changes in subependymal tissue in the demyelinating quaking animal.

Analysis of movement pattern supports evidence that the dominant syndrome in the staggerer is that of unopposed laybrynthine activity. Clinical characteristics of the quaking mice have been established and the date of appearance of seizures appears to be nutritionally related. Animals with special diet do not develop seizures until later dates. Electrical analysis of these animals is continuing. A new cerebellar mutant, nervous specimen is being studied because of its relative Purkinje cell degeneration.

A set of staggerers and quaking mice are being subjected to L-Dopa medication to see whether this will modify to some degree fixed postures, tremulousness, and ataxias. Perfection of perfusion techniques for better fixation of specimens and embedding continues.

Because of the lack of EM support, and time to be able to continue to carryout this study, no further observations have been made. Nonetheless, the colony of effected mice has been maintained. Further data is being collected on the aging phenomenon as related to the animals with this disorder.

SUPPORTED BY:
U.S. Veterans Administration

ROLE OF PYRUVATE CARBOXYLASE IN METABOLIC REGULATION,
M.C. SCRUTTON, Temple University, School of Medicine, Philadelphia, Pennsylvania 19122

Pyruvate carboxylases will be purified from brain and adipose tissue. The brain and adipose tissue enzymes will be characterized to determine whether the catalytic and regulatory properties differ from those observed from the enzyme in liver and reflect the anaplerotic (brain) and lipogenic/glyceroneogenic (adipose tissue) roles of the enzyme in these tissues. Pyruvate carboxylase will also be purified from the livers of rats and guinea pigs subjected to (1) dietary manipulations which might alter the relative contributions of the gluconeogenic and lipogenic contributions to the overall pyruvate yields oxalacetate flux and (2) physiological stresses (e.g. adrenalectomy, diabetes, starvation, exercise, ageing) which might also affect the relative contributions to the overall flux (especially for gluconeogenesis). Maximal catalytic capacities for pyruvate carboxylase will be determined in these various states.

The regulatory properties of pyruvate carboxylases in invertebrates and lower vertebrates will be examined to clarify the evolutionary relationships of these properties and hence to provide some indication of their physiological significance.

Studies will be conducted using denaturing conditions and group- specific reagents to probe the structural requirements for the interaction of pyruvate carboxylase from rat liver with its metabolic effectors (acetyl-CoA and L-malate). These studies are intended to clarify the mechanism (s) by which these effectors modify the catalytic activity of this pyruvate carboxylase.

SUPPORTED BY:
U.S. Dept. of Hlth. Ed. & Wel. - N.I.H.

PROCESS OF AGING IN THE CENTRAL NERVOUS
SYSTEM OF MICE,

S.S. SEKHON, U.S. Veterans Administration,
Hospital, Long Beach, California 90801

Our basic theme is to study the process
of aging in various areas of the CNS of
mice. The following two aspects of the
above problem were emphasized during the
past year: (1) Age-dependent changes in the
cervical anterior horn cells and (2) Delayed
effects of total body radiation on the
neurons of cerebral cortex.

The main structural changes observed in
the cervical anterior horn cells included
progressive increase of lipofuscin,
hypochromidia, and degradation of the Golgi
cisternae. Neurons with heavy deposits of
lipofuscin generally contained fewer
mitochondria, Nissl bodies, neurofilaments,
etc. Sequential events accompanying the
development of lipofuscin granules were
followed. Our results show that mature
lipofuscin granules evolve through
structural alterations of lysosomes. Initial
onset of pigmentation was first observed
within autophagic vacuoles. By accumulating
increasing amounts of residue, the
autophagic vacuoles eventually become
transformed into mature pigment granules of
complex substructure.

The cerebral cortex used in the
radiation study was obtained from
six-week-old animals which had been
administered 100 rads of total body
radiation at the age of three weeks. Extent
of radiation injury varied considerably;
some neurons appeared quite normal whereas
others showed extensive damage.
Vesiculation of cytoplasm, swelling and
disruption of endoplasmic reticulum,
disarray of mitochondrial cristae, changes
in mitochondrial matrix and clumping of

nuclear chromatin were the chief
manifestations of radiation injury. Our
future plans include continuation of the
study of the effects of varying doses of
radiation on different areas of the CNS, and
aging changes in neuroglia and synapses.

SUPPORTED BY:
U.S. Veterans Administration

AGING IN CONNECTIVE TISSUE, BRAIN AND THE
AUDITORY SYSTEM,
F.M. SINEX, Boston University, School of
Medicine, Boston, Massachusetts 02215

     The objectives of our Program Project
are to expand our studies of aging. To
provide a coherent framework for these
studies, the program has been restricted to
connective tissue, the brain and the
auditory system. There are eight individual
projects under four project directors. The
departments participating are Biochemistry,
Anatomy and Psychology.
     Our interdisciplinary studies will use
techniques as diverse as electron
microscopy, studies of circular dichroism
and operant conditioning. We hope to learn
essential information about the aging brain
and the relationship of biochemical,
morphological and behavioral change during
age.
     A variety of tissues will be used
throughout the course of our investigations.
 These include fibroblasts, smooth muscle
and neuronal elements in culture; and in the
central nervous system, the neocortex and
the olfactory bulbs.

SUPPORTED BY:
U.S. Dept. of Hlth. Ed. & Wel. - N.I.H.

FATTY ACID METABOLISM IN BRAIN SUBCELLULAR
MEMBRANES,
G.Y. SUN, Cleveland Psychiatric Inst.,
Cleveland, Ohio 44109

It has been increasingly recognized
that the normal metabolic processes of brain
components can be altered significantly by
neurological diseases, aging, and dietary
deficiencies. The main objectives of this
proposal are: (1) to study the metabolism of
fatty acids at the subcellular level of the
mouse brain, (2) to correlate fatty acid
metabolism in vivo in the brain of the
rodents to that of the primates, (3) to
examine the composition of brain lipids in
mouse and in human autopsies with age, (4)
to compare the metabolism of brain membrane
lipids in mice with known dietary
deficiencies, and (5) to study the
metabolism of membrane lipids in mouse brain
at various intervals during development,
maturation and aging.
     C14-labeled long chain fatty acids (
16:0, 18:0, 18:1, 18:2, 18:3 and 20:4) will
be injected intracerebrally into mice. At
selected periods after injection, animals
will be sacrificed and the brain will be
homogenized in 0.32M sucrose and subjected
to subcellular fractionation procedure.
Lipids will be extracted from the isolated
fractions by chloroform-methanol 2:1 (v/v).
Phospholipids will be analyzed by TLC and
the non-polar side chains will be converted
to their derivatives and analyzed by GLC.
Incorporation of the labeled precursors into
individual phospholipids, galactolipids and
neutral glycerides will be examined and
correlated.
     The long-term goal for this project is
to study the metabolism of fatty acids in
the mammalian brain membranes in an attempt
to relate possible variances with regard to
aging and various nutritional deficiences.

SUPPORTED BY:
U.S. Dept. of Hlth. Ed. & Wel. - N.I.H.

CYTOLOGIC STUDIES IN DISEASES OF THE NERVOUS
SYSTEM,
R.D. TERRY, Yeshiva University, School of
Medicine, Bronx, New York 10461

The major goal of this project is the
understanding of the pathogenesis and the
pathophysiology of age changes in the human
cerebrum. Our several approaches are based
on our past studies of the ultrastructure of
the senile plaque and neurofibrillary
tangle. Various animal models are being
studied in order to get at the separate
aspects of these lesions. Systemic
amyloidosis will be induced in mice and then
brain injuries will be created to see
whether and how focal amyloid deposits will
be formed in the brain. Organized neuronal
tissue cultures will be treated with iron
compounds to see whether the neurofibrillar
protein can be changed by means of this
oxialuminum treatment, and axoplasmic flow
will be measured relative to these
particular neurons. The ratio between
filaments and tubules in peripheral axons
will be altered by systemic treatment with
acrylamide, and axoplasmic flow will be
correlated with these changed ratios. Light
and electron microscopic studies will
continue of aged animal brains, especially
of primates whenever they can be obtained.

SUPPORTED BY:
U.S. Dept. of Hlth. Ed. & Wel. - N.I.H.

CLINICAL AND EEG EFFECTS FOLLOWING HYDERGINE
ADMINISTRATION,
B.J. WILDER, U.S. Veterans Administration,
Hospital, Gainesville, Florida 32601

Purpose of Study: To evaluate the
effects of Hydergine vs. Placebo on the EEG
and symptomatology of geriatric patients
suffering from cerebrovascular insufficiency
(CVI).

Theoretical Background: Previous
investigators have shown that Hydergine
(Sandoz) improves cerebral circulation and
enhances cerebral oxygen uptake in geriatric
patients suffering from chronic
cerebrovascular disease. Animal experiments
have demonstrated improved neuronal
metabolism. These studies also showed
"normalization" of the abnormal EEG within
the framework of these experiments.
Furthermore, in clinical situations,
Hydergine treated patients showed
improvement of certain CNS symptoms
attributed to chronic CV disease. Since the
EEG may be regarded as an index of cerebral
metabolism, it seems logical that clinical
trial of this drug be obtained in sampled
patients and the EEG records obtained will
be compared with the clinical changes.

Material and Methods: Forty hospital
patients,55 years of age or over, with
previous history of CVI (per selected
criteria) and a focal CVA 4-15 weeks prior
to inclusion in study, will be selected.
Study drug will be administered for 6 weeks,
at a daily dose of 6 (six) tablets
(Hydergine sublingual, marked by the sponsor
and matching Hydergine placebo tablets-
given at random). Neurological, mental, and
general physical examinations will be
carried out at weeks 0, 3, and 6 of the
study together with EEG, EKG, and blood
chemistry. The changes in each modality

will be compared as well as correlation
between the different criteria and between
the placebo and the drug receiving patients.
Results of this pilot study should indicate
the effectiveness of the drug, in this
homogenous group.

SUPPORTED BY:
U.S. Veterans Administration